The Real Life Stories Of Sickle Cell A Global Collaboration

Copyright © Agnes Nsofwa, Maureen Malama & Solome Mealin 2023

All rights reserved. No part of this book may be used, replicated or reproduced in any manner whatsoever without the author's written permission except for quotations of not more than 25 words which are solely for critical articles or reviews. Although the author and publisher have made every effort to ensure that the information in this book is correct at the time of printing, the author and publisher do not assume and, therefore, disclaim liability to any party. The author and the publisher will not be held responsible for any loss or damage, same for that caused by their negligence. Although the author and the publisher have made every reasonable attempt to achieve accuracy in the content of this book, they assume no responsibility for errors or omissions. You should only use this information as you see fit. Any use is at your own risk. You must act responsibly and sensibly in using the information, and your life and circumstances may not be suited to the examples shared within these pages. How you choose to include this information in this book within your own life is completely your own responsibility and at your own risk.

Published in 2023 by Olana's World Publishing House Olana's World Publishing House Melbourne Australia

https://agnesnsofwa.com.au

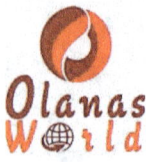

Table of Contents

Acknowledgement..7

Feedback From the Book Editor..........................9

Introduction...11

Queen Mother as A Sickle Cell Warrior - by - THE LATE MS MAUREEN MWEWA MALAMA AGNES' MOTHER..19

From The Eyes of a Warrior - by - DONNA ACHIENG...23

My Advice to Sickle Cell Warriors - by - DR ROBERT SOKOLIC..40

Sickle Cell Disease Memory's Story - by - EMELDA MULENGA...56

How Sickle Cell Disease Impacted My Family by - ESNART CHUSHI...61

Survival Journey from Sickle Cell by - ESTHER NGOMA..70

From Patient to Advocate - by - EUNICE OWINO.79

Sickle Cell Warrior - by - IGNATIUS MULENGA KABWE...97

Living With Sickle Cell: A Story of Strength - by - JOSEPH MUBANGA...111

My Sickle Cell Challenges Journey - by - K W YOUNG..….....124

My Journey with Sickle Cell and The Fight for Better Healthcare in Nigeria - by - OLUWAKEMI OGUNTIMEHIN……………………………..……..132

A Sickle Cell Journey of Hope and Resilience - by - AGNESS CHITAMBI………………………………161

Fighting The Silent Battle: A Story of a Warrior - by - LILLIAN CHIKUTA………………………….176

Aging Sickle Cell Patients. By - LINDA ARMSTEAD…………………………………....…..183

Sickle Cell And Me: Challenges Battle with Silent Disease - by - LUSUBILO GONDWE……….………191

Sickle Cell: A Journey of Hope and Strength - by - MNGURE DAISY……………………………………..204

How Sickle Cell Has Impacted Me - by - PATRICIA CHILESHE……………………………………….209

My Sickle Cell Trait Journey by - PHOSTINA MWANSA………………………………………….217

Sickle Cell Disease in Australia and Zambia A Comparison of The Two Countries I Call Home - by - AGNES NSOFWA…………………………………….234

The Comparison of Sickle Cell Care Between Uganda and The United Kingdom - by - SOLOME MEALIN……………………………………………..261

A Mother's Journey with Sickle Cell Disease and The Power of Community Support and The Need to Change Mindset - by - SYLVIA BWALYA MWANSA……..276

Sickle Cell Journey: From Struggles to Empowerment - by - VERAH NAMBAYA…………………………..292

The Sickle Cell Warrior - by - WEGGINESS MWANDILA…………………………………………..299

Sickle Cell Disease- by - ZAKAREYA ALKADHEM.319

Conclusion…………………………………..………326

References…………………………………………...328

Acknowledgement

As I sat down to read all these stories from these wonderful people from different parts of the world, my first thoughts were gratitude. Gratitude for having this privilege to be the one to tell these stories to the world. When my daughter was diagnosed with SCD in November 2019, little did I know the journey that I was going to go through all in the name of SCD. My journey has been interesting, although scary at times and being vulnerable most times, I thank the higher being for choosing me to tell these stories on behalf of different people from different countries.

Volume two of the SCD stories has not been well for me. In the middle of putting these stories together, I lost my greatest supporter of my SCD advocacy work. In the early hours of June 4th, 2023, my dear mum Maureen passed away alone, and this breaks my heart every day. A few days after her passing, I was numb, I could not think, I had so many questions and regrets. The most regret to today is why we left out home country and had to live 20 years without being in the same country with our dear mother. I wish I could have done things differently but after giving it a lot of thought and looking at different perspectives, I realised life is a mystery and we are all going to go one day. What differs is our different exit plan. I miss my mum every day and four months on, I still laugh at the fact that my mother is no more, it still doesn't make sense to me.

I want to take this opportunity to thank all mothers out there. You love us unconditionally and sometimes we may take it for granted that you will live forever. For caregivers of different warriors, thank you for all you do. You are the greatest gift to your children.
I dedicate this book to my mother Maureen Mwewa Malama Banda as she used to call herself. Rest in eternal peace mum, until we meet again. I love you more each day.

I would also like to dedicate this book to my husband Preston Nsofwa who is forever supporting me in everything that I do. His support makes me keep going even when it's difficult. His encouragement no matter each situation makes me the best version of myself. Thank you, Preston.

To my children, all four of you, thank you for being patient with me. I know I maybe the busiest mum at times but thank you for your continued support and for being patient with me. I love you from the moon and back.

To everyone reading this book, thank you. These stories are for you. I hope you get encouraged, inspired, and empowered in your own community to shine the light on sickle cell disease.

Agnes MN

Feedback from the Book Editor

We would like to include this piece from the book editor Patricia who sums up this book beautifully:

This is one of the best written complied stories that evoke empathy, sympathy, sadness, pains, and a sign of hope for all sickle cell patients. The stories of the patients and guardians were well narrated while addressing relevant issues affecting one's health.

The compelling collection of stories that artfully narrate the experiences of individuals living with sickle cell disease. This anthology not only sheds light on the challenges faced by those with sickle cell but also serves as a powerful testament to the indomitable spirit and resilience of these individuals. The publication's numerous reports offer a heartbreaking and enlightening glimpse into the daily lives, hardships, and victories of sickle cell sufferers.

The anthology's sincerity and raw passion make each tale a genuinely engaging and instructive read. The writers expertly express the physical and emotional toll of living with a chronic illness while also emphasizing the resilience and courage required to live with sickle cell.

The book's diversity of opinions is one of its most notable qualities. Each narrative is unique, providing a distinct perspective on the complexities of sickle cell disease.

The book not only teaches readers about sickle cell disease, but it also encourages empathy and understanding. It dismantles assumptions and misunderstandings, replacing them with a great appreciation for the tenacity of sickle cell patients.

Readers are encouraged to walk into the shoes of the narrators through the pages of this book, getting vital insights into the obstacles they confront and the resilience that keeps them going. The writers provide a vivid picture of the highs and lows that come with the territory of sickle cell illness, from victory to despair.

Introduction

It's 2023 and we are still noticing the challenges that people living with Sickle Cell Disease (SCD) go through. In this life of social media where everyone knows what others are experiencing, it has made so easy for all of us impacted by SCD to know what challenges different communities are going through.

The Real-Life Stories of Sickle Cell - A Global Collaboration is a book that brings out the lived experiences of different people living with SCD from different parts of the world. Our intention is for us to make the world understand the lives of those living with this disease. Through storytelling, we want health professionals, policymakers, politicians, Carers, and the whole world to know what people with SCD go through on a day today basis. Although these are individual stories, we hope by sharing this to the world, those who for any reason cannot share their stories maybe reminded that they are not alone.

SCD is the most common genetic disorder in the world but has received little attention. SCD affects any race, age, gender and as such, we should continue to break the myths and conceptions that SCD is a black disease. People with this condition may feel alone in many ways because no one understands what they are going through. This ends up being a lonely and sad journey in life as can be seen in different scenarios across this book.

The stories in this book are from people from all over the world, but we would like to highlight the story of a very strong lady who cannot pen the words down right now as she went to meet the Lord in June this year (2023), Mama Maureen Mwewa Malama (RIP). The very few words she told her daughter Agnes about SCD, represent the understanding of many, if not all parents especially those in less resource countries.

These stories are here to inspire people impacted by SCD the world over. Our hope is that these stories will contribute towards breaking the barriers that those with SCD to have a voice. In addition, we hope that those impacted by SCD and struggling to understand some challenges will get the help they need without being labelled or stigmatised.

As we continue to do our part to tell our stories, we remember many sickle cell warriors who have passed on without having to pen down their experiences. Through these stories, those who are not with us are, in one way or another, we hope their stories are represented, and we will continue to shine the candle for them.

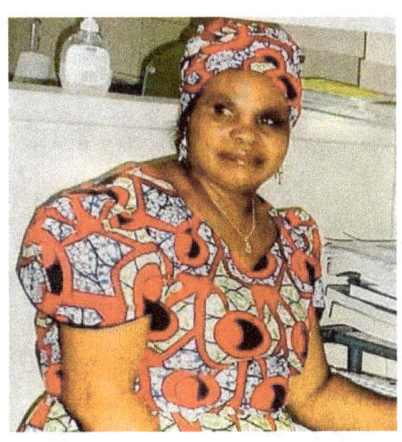

Queen Mother as a Sickle Cell Warrior
By the Late Ms Maureen Mwewa Malama
(Agnes' Mother)

I became aware I had the sickle cell trait when I was 23, during my pregnancy with Agnes, my first child, in the late 70s. Despite being a strong and healthy young woman without any signs of sickling, the turning point in my life was during my first antenatal check-up when the blood test showed a positive sickle cell trait. At that time, I disregarded the results without consulting the nurses, confident in my well-being even though I did not know about sickle cell. Subsequently, on October 24th, I gave birth without complications. It was a time of celebration, and Agnes, born on Independence Day, received gifts from Johnson and Johnson, alongside a Birth Certificate.

Throughout her early days in Chingola, spanning the first month and a few weeks, Agnes remained a happy and healthy child, seldom crying due to her constant thumb-sucking habit that persisted through her teenage years.

At that time, I worked as a Senior Collector at Income Tax, while her father held the position of Senior Inspector, a role that has since transitioned to ZRA. Remarkably, he was not a carrier of the Sickle Cell trait. Agnes never portrayed any signs and symptoms of this sickle cell disease; however, when she was 6 months old, she encountered her first significant illness—Measles. Though her body was covered in a rash, as a young mother, I did not recognize the ailment.

Agnes started her education journey at a Nursery School in Chingola, growing fast. When she turned 5, I wanted her to join Grade 1. Unfortunately, her being 5 years old resulted in her application being denied due to age. The outcome might have differed if she had been born earlier in the year. Despite this delay, Agnes displayed all the qualities of a Grade 1 student—bright, intelligent, strong, and fearless. She continued her education in Nursery School.

Agnes still displayed exceptional educational strength all through her nursery school. When Agnes reached the age of 7, it was then that she finally embarked on her Grade 1 journey in Chingola. Subsequently, she ventured to Lusaka and later to Chipata, culminating her academic journey with G12 completion at Chipata Day Secondary School. Interestingly, throughout these years, no signs of Sickle Cell manifested in Agnes, and I refrained from seeking advice from medical professionals about its implications. My other children are carriers of the trait but do not suffer from the disease, a fortunate outcome.

Joy, Agnes' child, significantly catalysed my extensive understanding of Sickle Cell. Born in September late 2000s, during my visit to Perth, a severe episode transpired. Agnes fell gravely ill during her 32-week pregnancy, and her blood levels declined precariously. Following numerous tests, a Sickle Cell Trait diagnosis was seen, accompanied by jaundice, and swelling. I realized I had unknowingly passed on this trait inherited from my late father, John.

Upon my return, I consulted her doctors, who wrestled with the challenge of administering medication due to Agnes' adverse reactions. Their counsel was to discontinue medication, place the Holy Bible beneath her pillow, and seek divine intervention through prayers led by her father, a priest. We engaged in fervent intercession; The Reverend and I prayed to God tirelessly for a month, forsaking rest, food, and sleep. Ultimately, our pleas were answered.

When I decided to end my fast, Agnes called home to tell us of her discharge and good health. My gratitude to God overflowed for saving her life and enlightening us about the seriousness of

Sickle Cell Disease. All glory to God. Today, Agnes has evolved into a global Sickle Cell Advocate and Consultant. May God bless her good heart.

NB: This story was contributed by my mother in January 2023. My mother died unexpectedly on 4th June 2023. I will forever cherish the woman that she was. Very supportive of all that I did. We sometimes take life for granted and I did not see Mum dying at such a young age and crucial time when we were planning for her to come and stay with us in Australia. But ultimately, we are all on this earth on borrowed time. All we can do and thank God for making it possible for us to share life with her. Continue resting in peace Mum, until we meet again. **Agnes Nsofwa, your daughter.**

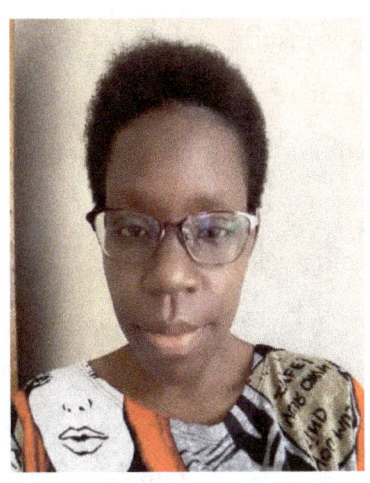

From the Eyes of a Warrior
By Donna Achieng

Early Childhood

My name is Donna Achieng. I was born and raised in Nairobi, Kenya. I am thirty- five years old. I have two brothers and I am the eldest. I had a very normal African childhood. The running in the rains, walking/ running long distances to school, having to face the wrath of some teachers due to failed tests, unfinished assignments or even just being late, playing till it's dark without sweaters, running around bare-footed; playing with mud, tadpoles, insects and small reptiles of all kinds, playing rough and high-intensity games like wrestling and so many other activities that took all the energy out of me, my siblings and our friends.

Weirdly enough, most of the above activities should have made me prone to infections or crises but alas!!! I was quite ok all through. In my early years, my parents never knew I had Sickle Cell Anaemia.

The only sign I had was just the yellow eyes but when we went to the doctor, the only thing he recommended was that I take more carrots and glucose and I will be ok. I guess my parents never thought so much about it and they never saw the need to investigate further the cause of my eyes turning yellow, or like my fellow students referred to them, "green eyes". Why would they anyway, I was ok health-wise, I did not have any ailments or complications, I was always active and rarely fell sick. No cause for alarm! The 'green eyes' started bothering many students and when it reached that point, I would be sent home to go get checked. As usual, I would be given carrots and lots of water and few days later, my eyes would be clearer, and I would be back to school. This was the norm for the fifteen years I lived without knowing I had Sickle Cell Anaemia.

My parents later passed away in 2002 without ever knowing about my health status, (or maybe they knew but hid it from everyone including me, this we shall never know). After my father's funeral, I developed a wound on my right foot. No one was concerned and after a month, it disappeared by itself. I guess that was my very first encounter with a leg *ulcer*.

Boarding School Life and First Diagnosis

In 2003, I joined high school. My nickname there was 'last born' because I had a very small physique compared to my fellow classmates. I was in a boarding school, in a new environment, far away from home. I and my brothers now lived with our guardians who were our relatives. The first two terms were quite ok. I did what every student in a typical Kenyan boarding school does. I attended all classes including the very early morning preps and night preps too, bathed with cold water all through my entire four years there, ate meals that every other student ate; no special meals maybe in the case of allergies, and did my duties like everyone else. These duties included cleaning classrooms and dormitories, sweeping the school compound and picking rubbish, washing the corridors and toilets, bathrooms and dining area, fetching water from boreholes or rivers when it ran out, and cleaning the serving dishes used in the dining hall. I did all that without any problems. I even wore uniforms that were not properly dried because sometimes we got our uniforms stolen by the older students so one ends up having to wash the remaining uniform, they still had daily. Bad luck if the weather was not favourable, you had to wear them when damp the next day. I am still surprised this also never affected me.

Later still in my first year of high school, we had no water and we all had to go to the nearest river/ borehole to bring some for our own use. I found some in a borehole so did not have to go to the river. I carried my bucket full of water on my head. I had learnt to do this in school. I had done it severally, but this day was different. I could even remove it from my head all by myself but on this day, I had no strength. I asked a friend to help me put it down, but she took her time because she was eating. I had to wait for her to go wash her hands and come help me. My body couldn't handle it any longer and the next thing I knew, I woke up in the school nurse's office. I was not feeling sick, just fatigued. She got worried and took me to a hospital outside our school. The hospital did not have many facilities, so I was referred to a bigger hospital. My guardian was called to come and take me to the hospital. He came the next day and off we went. Both I and he agreed that this was just a waste of time because I was fine, even the fatigue had faded off. All the same, we went, and the required tests were carried out. Two weeks later, the results were back, and it was official. I had Sickle Cell Anaemia. I was sixteen years old. I had no idea what that was or how serious it was. My uncle too was confused. He had not heard of such a condition in our family history and wondered where I got it from. We all thought and believed it came from my mother's side. A sad reality of how much awareness was needed back then and still needed now. The doctor did not elaborate much too, the only thing we were told was that I was going to be taking medicine every day for the rest of my life.

I went back to school. I was neither worried nor full of questions. I was just my normal self. If only I knew of the severity of this condition... I continued with my normal boarding school routine except for taking part in vigorous activities. Though once in a while, a teacher who did not understand my condition did put me through vigorous exercise and if I did not participate, I was punished. I continued bathing with cold water, too. The only thing that got to me was when my schoolmates started telling me how they had heard that people living with this condition would never see their eighteenth birthday. I made peace with the fact that I had just two more years on earth. I will soon be joining my parents anyway. I went for regular check-ups as recommended and took my meds too. That was also the first time I was put on **hydroxyurea.** The leg ulcer recurred a year later and this made me go for dressing every few days. Good thing it only lasted for two months. I have never had another case of leg ulcer since 2004.

All through my high school, the only 'serious' issue I had, apart from the leg ulcer, was passing out and nothing else. Luckily for me, the passing outs mostly happened when I was at home and not in school. Another thing I also noticed was, that I still looked like a small girl, unlike my classmates who had started looking like beautiful young women. I had no hips, small breasts, no pimples on my face and I definitely had not yet started seeing my periods. I was never worried about all these; I still led a normal life. I got done with my high school without ever experiencing the above mentioned.

When my Death Day's had been Decided

Something worth noting is when 2005 came, I started preparing myself mentally because I knew I would soon be eighteen and my death day was fast approaching. The more August 30th approached, the more anxious I became. I believed everyone who told me I would not see my eighteenth birthday. The day came and I could not even sleep. The torments were too much. I finally fell asleep and hours later, woke up to the awesome discovery I was not dead! I was NOT DEAD!! I whispered a prayer and continued with my day, my birthday, with no more stress. When we opened school in September, I walked majestically into our school compound because I was back there to prove my naysayers wrong. I was alive and God had seen me through the past years. I had no complications too. I thought I was done with their mockery but alas!!! They were back to hit the nail on the head. I was again told that as much as I had seen my eighteenth birthday, I was among the very few lucky ones and that I should brace myself for my upcoming death when I turned twenty- two. Seems I would never catch a break from the death threats from these people. This time around, I had a little faith in me. I turned eighteen and I was ok, I will surely see my twenty-second birthday. I went on with my high school life until I completed my fourth year.

First Encounter with a Person Going Through a Crisis

It reached a time when I had to stop going for regular check-up's due to lack of finances. I was still not feeling unwell, so it did not bother me. I completely stopped taking my routine meds too. On my last check-up, I came across a certain lady crying like a baby. She looked like she was in her 40s. I asked my doctor what was up with the woman, and he told me if I had ever experienced a crisis. Never had I ever heard of it and he told me the day, I will get one then I will know why the lady was screaming in pain. The moment I left the hospital, I had forgotten about her and her screams. That was the last time I was in that hospital. Life moved on smoothly and I got done with high school in 2006.

College Life

In 2007, I was mostly indoors. I was an introvert so never really interacted with many people. This is the year I got my first period. I was twenty but looked like a fifteen-year-old. They mostly came for a day or two and then disappeared until the next month. At times a month or two went by without me having my menses. This was the year too I was taken to an herbalist who gave me some weird seeds, charcoal, citric and turmeric to be taking. I was still not unwell in any way, I still took them religiously, but I did not feel any change in my body. Things went on smoothly too and by the time the year was ending, I was to join college. When I did, as usual, I was the smallest among them all. I was ok with it. I had embraced my small physique and I loved it. College was fun but because I was an introvert, I never really got to go all out when it came to experiencing college life to the fullest. I have never smoked; I have gone out clubbing till the wee hours of the morning very few times, I have tasted alcohol and still, I was never affected in anyway way. During those days, I ate quite a lot of junk food too.

First Pain Episode

The year that changed my perception of Sickle Cell Anaemia was 2008. I was hanging out with a friend in a certain park. We were just chilling and catching up, enjoying the scenery. We were seated on the grass and about two hours into our meeting, I started feeling numb in my arms. We both thought that maybe if we changed our sitting position maybe, just maybe the numbness would wear off. It did subside but about fifteen minutes later, the numbness came back in my legs too. We decide to stand up and stretch a bit then take a short stroll around. This time around, the numbness persisted. Instead of subsiding, it started spreading all over my body. The meet-up came to an end as my friend proposed we postpone it to the next day and that I go rest. I concurred. Another mistake I made was to walk back to my hostel instead of taking a cab or public transport.

I could not have known otherwise; I would have taken precautions. This could have saved me and maybe prevented the 'numbness' from spreading. We walked about an hour and a half together with my friend who made sure I arrived safely. I decided to take a nap thinking I was just tired after the day's activities. A while later, I could not sleep because I had started feeling pain in my fingertips. It was not severe, so I decided to try and go back to sleep. That is when all hell broke loose. The pain spread so fast all over my body and I was now screaming and writhing in pain. My roommate came running and I told her what was happening. She is among the few who knew about my health condition. She gathered up a few other ladies and they carried me to the nearest pharmacy/ clinic to get help but being a weekend, all of them were closed.

The other option was another small local health centre that was some distance away and they had to cross a busy highway with them carrying me like a log. I was still screaming. The pain got worse when either one of the ladies pulled on my leg or the other pulled my arm. I was crying and wishing for death. This pain was nothing like I had experienced before. We attracted so much attention from passers-by and people in vehicles all around us. About twenty minutes later, they arrived with me at the hospital, and I just heard the attending nurse ask them what had happened to me and they said I just started screaming saying I was in pain. She ran inside and came back with an injection; I do not know what was in that syringe. A moment later before she injected me, she asked if any of the ladies who had brought me knew anything about me and if I had any underlying condition.

My roommate told her I had Sickle Cell and she stopped right in her tracks. I shouted for her to please take away the pain, but I heard her tell them I needed to get to an emergency room immediately or they would lose me. One of the ladies called a taxi and immediately, I was rushed to the nearest public hospital. I had not even realized that this was a crisis. One of the ladies accompanied me to the hospital. When we arrived, I was put on IV and moments later, I kind of drifted away into slumber land. It was at night now and I guess my body had been through so much. A few hours later, I woke up feeling ok but the doctors and nurses decided to admit me just to keep a close eye on me. My friend left but made sure I was comfortable and that she had informed my family. I will forever be grateful to these amazing ladies for their help and support when I needed it most. The next day, the doctors told me I experienced a crisis and was put under surveillance in the hospital for a whole month. That is the longest I have ever been in hospital and that is what my first ever crisis put me through. After that, I have been having severe crises less and less. Most times, I just experience mild ones that I can manage at home. I now know why that lady was crying her heart out. A crisis is something I would never wish on anyone, not even my worst enemy.

College life went on smoothly after that, nothing serious and never encountered that extreme crisis until much later in life. Left college and led a normal life with no serious issues, just mild pains and collapsing once in a while. I have never had leg ulcers again.

I got a few jobs here and there, nothing strenuous but I must admit I haven't had a decent job in a long while. I have lived with different relatives, especially after college and I am so grateful for them. I was well taken care of when I was going through the pains; the one thing that was a bit challenging was still the finances. One time, I was in so much pain and we had to just wait until we had borrowed money from friends and other relatives so that I could finally be taken to hospital. Most of the people I stayed with, were impoverished so it was hard when I was unwell. And none of us had a job.

In 2013, I decided to start living alone and see what life had in store for me. All was ok, had family and friends checking up on me every now and then. I did everything for myself be it house chores or running errands around or far. I was fine. I remember I used to carry 20 litre jerry cans full of water from the ground floor to 2nd floor without any hitches; I could also wash my duvets by myself and hang them without any help. I ate anything and everything too; I honestly never concentrated on a balanced diet. I ate whatever was available. I still hadn't gone for my routine check-ups or had my routine meds for years. I could not afford it. I only had pain meds that I took occasionally when in pain.

Pregnancy and Sickle Cell

I and my partner have known each other since 2008. He is a pharmacist and has been of great help when I am down health-wise. Some people were against our relationship because of my health status. He was told it was not a good idea because he would exhaust all his money and remain with nothing treating me, we were told I would never give birth and even if I did, I would die in the process or I would give birth to dead babies. This was too much to handle but we stood our ground. I am grateful for him standing by me all through these torments.

In late 2014, we discovered I was pregnant. I had felt my skin become so smooth and missed my periods but that was not a surprise because it was normal for me to miss them for even three months. The smoothness was what was weird. I assumed it for some time but when it persisted, we just had to carry out a test. I mostly have dry skin, so this was unusual. We found out I was expectant. My first thought was I am so DEAD!! This was because of the countless stories of me dying or giving birth to dead babies and because some people were against our relationship. We also had no stable jobs then. It took a toll on me. I had really wanted a baby but not under these circumstances. I had also not gone for a check-up for so long so I also became worried that I might not carry the pregnancy to term. We decided to not let our family and friends know until later. There were very few who knew. Some were not impressed because they said I was risking my life, and some were so happy for us.

I am amazed at how my pregnancy was smooth and without any problems. I ate everything, I took long walks without getting tired, and I still did my chores, though he helped every now and then. I only experienced a mild crisis during my 6th month and was admitted for two days. It was not serious, but the doctor was just taking extra precautions. I started my pre-natal clinics at 5 months. I neither visited a haematologist nor a gynaecologist. I went to the normal pre-natal clinics where the 'normal' pregnant women attended their clinics too. It never occurred to me that I needed a haematologist. I was still ok with my Hb ranging between 7 and 9.

On July 26th, I started experiencing the pains that came on and off. We first assumed they are the normal mild crisis or that my baby was playing too much in there. When it persisted, we called a nurse friend, and she told us I was in labour. We went to the hospital, and I got checked in. Most of the doctors and nurses did not believe I was in labour because I was just calm. I told them my crisis pain was worse than what I was experiencing at that moment and to me, a single sickle cell crisis is far much worse than going through labor. It was in the afternoon, and by the time it got to midnight, my passage hadn't fully opened, and I was told I would be undergoing a C-section because now my baby was in distress and my water had not broken too. I was later taken to the theatre and got my baby. My blood count was at 8 and I am surprised that I was not even transfused, and I was ok. Apart from inhaling a little amniotic fluid and a little jaundice, my baby was ok and she was taken to the New Born Unit. When I was able to walk, just a few hours later, I went to see her. I was walking around like someone who had not even gone through CS. I just cannot explain but I was not in so much pain. A few days later, we were discharged, and I beat the odds again. I have a beautiful daughter now and she is heaven-sent. She already knows a little about sickle cell and she knows what to do when I am unwell. I feel heartbroken when I cannot do stuff with her at times due to my health, but she understands. I make up for lost time whenever I can. I have been doing all my chores and still taking care of her without help from other people apart from my husband. Occasionally, I have had a few people help.

I also got my first ever transfusion in 2020 at 33 years of age when I decided I needed to just go and do an overall check-up; the doctor discovered my Hb was at 6.9 and immediately requested I do a transfusion. By then, my husband worked in a very nice private hospital and the hospital catered for the bills. In other circumstances that would have been so expensive. Since then, I have recently been to the hospital, where my blood count was tested, and it was the lowest ever at 5.6. Seeking treatment for us people with chronic conditions is so hard and due to unavoidable circumstances, we just sit out at home and pray we get better. Most of us resort to over-the-counter medicine to self-treat ourselves which is also dangerous. It is possible for warriors to do things that most people out there think we cannot. This is my story.

Conclusion

I have come to learn that all persons living with Sickle Cell Anaemia experience things differently. The intensity is different, the number of times we experience the pains is different, the number of hospitalizations, transfusions, complications arising from Sickle Cell, how we achieve our milestones from birth, pregnancy and every other aspect of our lives. Sometimes even the medications that work for one or routines might never work for another warrior. In all these, most of us have become aware of how our bodies work and how to go about taking care of our health. I have had a few issues that have come up due to having Sickle cell. These include/included leg ulcers,

Pica, gallstones, poor vision, frequent chest pains, jaundice, enlarged stomach, extreme fatigue, memory loss and a few more. Most days I am grateful to God for this far and truly I have reached a place where many warriors would have wished to reach but they could not. I hope my story will encourage even a single person out there.

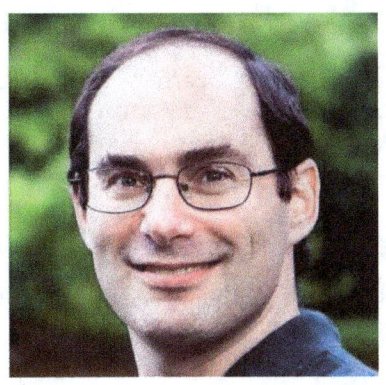

My Advice to Sickle Cell Warriors
By Dr Robert Sokolic

Sickle cell disease is an inherited disorder. Babies are born with the disease. No one chooses to have sickle cell disease, and no one should feel guilty or ashamed to have the illness. While most people with sickle cell disease are of African, South Asian, or Arabian descent, the disease can affect anyone. The gene that is affected in sickle cell disease is called *HGB*. The gene instructs the patient's red blood cells to make haemoglobin, the main protein in these cells. People with sickle cell disease have a type of haemoglobin protein called haemoglobin S. People without sickle cell disease typically have haemoglobin A

Red blood cells with haemoglobin S are stiffer than those of people who do not have sickle cell disease. The stiff red blood cells clog up the smallest blood vessels so that blood does not flow smoothly to all the organs and tissues in the body. The cells break down more quickly causing a low red blood cell count (anaemia). This blockage of blood flow and breakdown of red blood cells underlie all of the symptoms of sickle cell disease. Without treatment, Sickle cell disease can be severe and can lead to early death. With proper medical care, however, patients with sickle cell disease can live long and live well. There are three parts of good medical care for people with sickle cell disease, and these are the same as for people who do not have sickle cell disease. People with SCD need to live a healthful lifestyle, need to have regular primary and preventive care, and need to have compassionate medical treatment focused on their whole selves, including specific care for SCD.

Warriors should know their Genotype.

There are several genetic forms (genotypes) of sickle cell disease. Each person inherits two haemoglobin genes – one from the mother and one from the father. There are several unusual haemoglobin genes that can cause disease. A haemoglobin S gene is always present in people with sickle cell disease. If both the haemoglobin gene inherited from the mother and the haemoglobin gene inherited from the father are haemoglobin S genes, then the child has sickle cell anaemia. Another way to have sickle cell anaemia is to inherit one haemoglobin S gene from one parent and a gene for beta thalassemia major (called beta-nought thalassemia) from the other parent. Such a person also has sickle cell anaemia. If a person inherits a haemoglobin S gene and a gene for beta thalassemia minor (called beta-plus thalassemia), the person's disease is called sickle-beta-plus thalassemia. Another common haemoglobin abnormality is haemoglobin C. If a patient inherits one gene for haemoglobin S and one for haemoglobin C, the person has sickle haemoglobin C disease. There are other less common types of sickle cell disease genotypes. The reason why a warrior should know their genotype is to avoid misdiagnosis. I've had several patients who were told that they did not have sickle cell anaemia but were carriers of both sickle cell disease and beta-nought-thalassemia. This is incorrect. Such people have full-blown sickle cell anaemia, with all of the attendant risks and treatment implications.

There are several tests for sickle cell disease. The most common is a solubility test. One brand name for such a test is Sickledex. The sickle solubility test detects the presence of haemoglobin S but does not give any more information. So, a person who is a carrier of sickle trait, a person with sickle cell anaemia and a person with sickle haemoglobin C disease all have a positive result. More sophisticated tests for sickle cell disease include haemoglobin electrophoresis and high-performance liquid chromatography (HPLC). Ultimately, in difficult cases, DNA sequencing may be needed. For sickle cell warriors, the upshot is that one should know that at least the haemoglobin electrophoresis test has been done. If there is any concern that the clinical situation does not entirely match the supposed haemoglobin variant, more sophisticated testing, such as HPLC or comprehensive genetic testing of both alpha and beta globin genes should be performed. It may be difficult to locate a lab that does such testing, but the evaluation typically only has to be done once, so it is worthwhile to travel to a centre specializing in haemoglobin disorders if at all possible. Every doctor caring for sickle cell warriors should be able to tell the warriors their genotype. If the physician expresses that there is some uncertainty in the diagnosis, or if the clinical situation does not align with the diagnosis, additional testing should be done.

Until a complete genetic evaluation is done, there is always a possibility that something unusual is going on.

Healthy lifestyle for sickle cell warriors

A healthy lifestyle is recommended for all people, regardless of whether they have any identified medical illness. Even people who are quite sick do better with their illnesses if they are starting with a foundation of good health. In the USA, a healthy lifestyle involves eating a varied diet, getting appropriate exercise, and avoiding substances known to cause disease.

There are many types of diet that may be appropriate for people with sickle cell disease, but there are a few considerations that apply to everyone. A warrior's diet should be culturally appropriate. The diet should include lots of fruits and vegetables, and people with sickle cell disease should drink lots of water. While fruits and vegetables are important for everyone, they are particularly important for people with sickle cell disease because they contain high amounts of vitamin B9. This vitamin is also known as folate or folic acid. It is important for people with sickle cell disease to get a lot of folates because the vitamin is needed to make red blood cells. Because the red blood cells of people with sickle cell disease break down quickly, warriors need to make very many red blood cells and therefore need a lot of folate. While it is generally best to get nutrients from food rather than supplements, warriors need so much folate that it is almost always necessary for Warriors to take extra folate in the form of pills. Folate pills are very inexpensive and are widely available without a doctor's prescription. Even if a warrior is taking folate, eating a lot of fruits and vegetables brings many other health benefits.

Water is also an important nutrient for people with sickle cell disease. When the body is dehydrated, sickle cells are more likely to become very stiff and lead to painful crises and damage to organs. In a climate similar to the USA, I generally advise sickle cell warriors to drink at least two litters of water a day. More water is needed after vigorous exercise or on very hot days. A person can generally know that he or she is getting enough water if the urine is light yellow or clear. Darker urine indicates either not enough water or an impending sickle cell crisis.

Exercise is as important for sickle cell warriors as it is for other people. The US lifestyle is such that most US citizens do not get enough exercise just by doing their normal activities, and so have to exercise additionally on most days of the week. While this is important for people with sickle cell disease, there are some special considerations. People with sickle cell disease should exercise in moderation. When running, it is important to wear proper running shoes. The bones and joints can be fragile in sickle cell disease, and therefore more prone to injury. While exercising, it is important for people with sickle cell disease to increase their water intake, so as not to become dehydrated.

Finally, a healthy lifestyle includes avoiding substances that lead to ill health, such as alcohol, tobacco, or nicotine in any form and drugs of abuse. Where it is legal and culturally appropriate, people with sickle cell disease can use alcohol in moderation, such as 1 or two drinks per night one or two times a week. Warriors should avoid getting drunk as a lot of alcohol is dehydrating and when drunk people are more likely to suffer injury. There is no safe amount or type of tobacco or nicotine, and these substances should not be used by sickle cell warriors. With respect to drugs of abuse, there is only moderate agreement as to what substances fall into this category. For example, cocaine is generally thought to be quite risky for sickle cell disease with virtually no benefits to health. Marijuana is a special case in the USA. The drug remains illegal at the federal level, although there have been claims of benefit in certain medical conditions including sickle cell disease. While there is little evidence to support these claims, most states allow people with certain illnesses to use marijuana, and under the laws of some states, the drug is legal for any use. If warriors are going to use marijuana, smoking is the least preferable form, as smoking marijuana can cause the same types of lung diseases associated with smoking tobacco.

Primary and preventive care for sickle cell warriors

For all patients, having an ongoing relationship with a primary care provider whom one trusts and whom one sees when well is the foundation of good medical care. Many people with sickle cell disease see their haematologist (specialist in blood diseases) so frequently that they do not receive primary care, but this is not the best kind of medicine. Of course, in many parts of the world, there is no ready access to haematologists. However, there is no need for a warrior to get primary care from a haematologist. Any primary care provider, including non-physician providers such as nurse practitioners, can deliver appropriate wellness interventions and preventive medicine to sickle cell warriors, as they do to any other group of patients.

Preventive care and routine follow-up are cornerstones of good medical care for everyone and for sickle cell warriors. People with sickle cell disease can get any of the illnesses that people without SCD can get, and the effects of such illnesses can be more severe in a person with sickle cell disease in the background. Routine screening that is appropriate for the general population is therefore also appropriate for people with SCD. Amon preventive interventions, vaccination is even more important for people who have SCD than for people who do not because people who have SCD are often immune compromised. A primary care physician is also the type of doctor most used to coordinate complex care requiring the services of multiple specialists. People with SCD often fall into this category as they continue to age and suffer wear and tear from SCD. Finally, primary care providers are often more accessible than subspecialists. In addition to routine screening and preventive care, it is important to screen for and try to prevent or pre-empt complications of sickle cell disease. Screening should include blood and urine tests, eye exams and possibly other studies aimed at detecting problems in the lungs and heart.

Vaccination is critical for sickle cell warriors. Almost all people with sickle cell disease have immune deficiency because of damage to the spleen. This time of immune deficiency leaves warriors particularly vulnerable to severe outcomes from certain bacterial infections (called encapsulated organisms). Vaccination can prevent warriors from catching these infectious diseases. All sickle cell warriors are at risk for damage to their liver from sickle cell disease, and so immunization against various forms of hepatitis is also important. Finally, vaccinations that are indicated for everyone, such as those against flu and COVID-19, are especially important for sickle cell warriors, because these infections may be more severe in people with sickle cell disease than they are in people who do not have sickle cell disease.

It is essential to know one's primary care physician well so that he or she can recognize changes that may signal illness. Knowing a person well will also make it easier for the doctor to advocate for him or her when he or she is sick. The best way for a doctor to know a person well is for the doctor to see that person when he or she is healthy and at regular intervals.

Specialty care for Sickle Cell Warriors

While primary care is important, all people with SCD should also see a doctor or other provider with a specific interest in SCD. This does not need to be a haematologist. Any health care provider who wants to do so can learn to care for people with SCD. Special skills beyond standard medical training are not required. That being said, the majority of physicians with special interests in caring for people with

SCD are haematologists. Haematologists are often the doctors with the easiest access to some of the special interventions that may be of benefit to people with sickle cell disease, and some of the medicines used for SCD are most familiar to haematologists from their care of patients with other blood diseases.

If a warrior cannot routinely access a haematologist frequently, even a single meeting, or infrequent meetings can be very helpful. Certain lab tests that are ideal for the management of sickle cell disease are not carried out in regular clinical labs but can be accessed through a haematologist. While it is important to occasionally have such tests, they are not needed frequently. Everything that a warrior needs to fight SCD on a day-to-day basis is generally available at most labs. While some of the newer drugs used to treat SCD are very expensive or otherwise not available in all places, the most commonly needed medicines and procedures are widely available.

It is very often the case that other types of specialists are involved in the care of people with sickle cell disease because the disease can affect all parts of the body. Depending on how CD has affected a warrior, they may need to see doctors specialized in the care of the heart, the lungs, the kidneys or other organs. Surgeons may be required, although ideally any surgery is planned in conjunction with a warrior's sickle cell doctor. Specialists in symptom management, rehabilitation medicine, psychiatry and psychology may also be needed. If a warrior sees a number of different specialists, the care needs to be coordinated, such that one doctor's prescriptions don't interfere with those of another doctor. The ideal person to coordinate such care is a primary care physician, although haematologists may assume these responsibilities as well.

Treatments for Sickle Cell Disease

There are several treatments available for warriors. The first treatment is almost always aimed at treating symptoms, especially pain. Treating pain does not modify the course of the disease, but treats suffering and so, is mandatory. Treating pain and other symptoms, however, is not sufficient treatment in most cases, because treating the pain does not change the long-term course of the disease. In order to get the best outcomes, disease-modifying treatments almost always need to be given. The most well-known, least expensive and most efficacious disease-modifying treatment is hydroxyurea, the only medicine known to prolong the lives of people with sickle cell disease. Other disease-modifying medicines include crizanlizumab (Adakveo), which is given IV, and Voxelotor (Oxbryta), which is a pill. Folic acid in pill form is a foundation of sickle cell treatment, as noted above in the section on diet.

The problem with the disease-modifying medicines is that they work slowly. In the case of hydroxyurea, one must start at a low dose and build up the dose gradually. Because the dose is based on weight, building up to the right dose can take more than a year in heavier warriors. If warriors are not told that the medicines take time to work, they may stop taking the medicines too soon, and therefore miss out on the possibility of benefit. Also, physicians may decrease or stop pain medicines too soon without giving the disease-modifying medicines time to work.

This is one of the many reasons why communication between doctors and warriors is essential for good care for people with sickle cell disease.

The most straightforward treatment, at least conceptually, is blood transfusion, and there are several clinical situations where transfusion is indicated. Sometimes, just giving blood (simple transfusion) is enough. In other cases, sickle blood cells have to be removed and replaced by donor cells with the standard form of haemoglobin. This is called an exchange transfusion.

Finally, the ultimate cure for any disease of blood cells is bone marrow transplantation (also called stem cell transplant). Bone marrow is a tissue inside of a person's bones. It is the factory that makes blood cells. If a warrior is given the bone marrow of a person who does not have sickle cell disease, and if the treatment works as planned, the warrior will have won the war, and will no longer have sickle cell disease. Bone marrow transplant is not appropriate for everyone, as there are considerable up-front risks, including a realistic risk of death. Many warriors have been told that they cannot have a bone marrow transplant because they do not have a match. This was much more commonly the case in the past. Advances in bone marrow transplant in recent years, and the advent of umbilical cord blood transplant, have made it possible to use bone marrow from unrelated donors, or even half-matched donors to cure sickle cell disease, almost all warriors have an available half-matched donor because both parents are half-matched to their child. Certain aspects of a warrior's disease may make bone marrow transplantation inadvisable, including immunological reactions to previous blood transfusions, and complications of sickle cell disease that have damaged vital organs, but a discussion of bone marrow transplantation is always appropriate.

An alternative to using bone marrow from another person to cure sickle cell disease is to remove a warrior's own marrow, to correct the sickle cell mutation and to infuse the corrected marrow back into the warrior. This is called gene therapy. Several types of gene therapy have been tried in sickle cell warriors, but there have been some severe adverse outcomes, and the therapy still remains experimental. Nevertheless, gene therapy may soon become an approved and accepted treatment for sickle cell disease and may allow curative therapy without the need for a donor or the risks of bone marrow transplantation.

Not every weapon is appropriate for every warrior, but all available treatment options should be discussed with warriors, and the best choice selected by the warrior in collaboration with their health-care provider.

Partnering with Health Care Providers

Ultimately, the health of a sickle cell warrior can be optimized by working in partnership with one's health care providers. Both warrior and doctor bring knowledge to the doctor-warrior relationship, but the knowledge that they each bring is complementary.

Only a sickle cell warrior knows their symptoms. As a physician, I do not know the pain of a sickle cell crisis. I don't know what it's like to be considered to be "drug seeking." However, I do know that fever in a patient with SCD is a medical emergency. I know that taking hydroxyurea extends life. I know that when the tricuspid regurgitant jet increases above 2.5 meters per second the chance of dying increases dramatically, and that better control of SCD can decrease the chance of this happening. I can never know what my patients feel, but I have been trained to explain to them what I find on examination of their bodies and their blood, and what the implications of these findings are. Even so, my prognoses are only somewhat accurate. In any case, the choice of treatment is up to the patient. Only they know their own values and preferences. I've had patients whose choices shortened their lives and increased their pain. Sometimes they could explain why they chose as they did, and sometimes I could understand the choice. Even when I cannot understand their choices, I can respect them. When the physician respects what the patient knows and feels, and the patient respects what the physician finds and explains, the best health outcomes are most likely to occur.

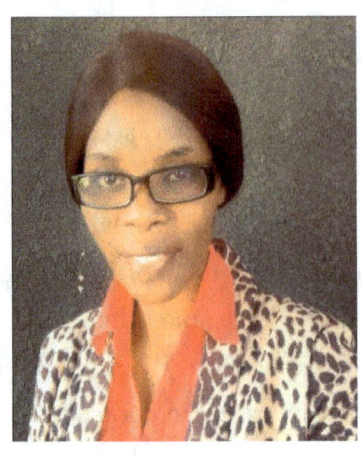

Sickle Cell Disease Memory's Story
By Emelda Mulenga

My name is Emelda Mulenga, am going to share with you my niece's sickle cell disease story or her sickle cell journey. Memory Mwansa is a young girl aged 8 years old and she is a sickle cell patient, Mwansa has lived with sickle cell disease or condition since she was born, though her parents discovered that she has sickle cell disease when Mwansa was 6 months old. But before I go into details, allow me to define sickle cell disease.

What is Sickle Cell Disease?

Sickle cell disease is a group of inherited red blood cell disorders that affects haemoglobin, the protein that carries oxygen through the body, the condition affects more than 100,000, people in the United States and 20 million people worldwide. Normally, red blood cells are disc-shaped and flexible enough to move easily through the blood vessels. If you have sickle cell disease, your red blood cells are present or sickle cell shaped, these cells do not bend or move easily and can block blood flow to the rest of your body.

The blocked blood flow through the body can lead to serious problems, including, stroke, eye problems, infections and episodes of pain called crisis. Sickle cell disease is a lifelong illness A blood and bone marrow transplant is currently the only the only cure for sickle cell disease, but there are effective treatments that can reduce the symptoms and prolong life. Your health care team will work with you on a treatment plan to reduce your symptoms and manage the condition. Without taking much of your time, allow me to go straight to the main point of writing my niece's story. It all started when Mwansa was born, her screening results showed that she had the most severe form of SCD, Sickle cell anaemia.

Sickle cell anaemia happens when two sickle cell genes are inherited, one from each parent. When Mwansa's mother first got the news, it was just one of those things that she thought she would just need to follow up with, she didn't know much about it until when Mwansa was 6 months old, she experienced her first severe pain episode. Her hands and joints were swollen, and Mwansa kept on crying and her mother didn't know what to do because she didn't know what was wrong with the child. So, she took Mwansa to the hospital and the doctors told her that Mwansa was experiencing a pain episode which occurs when sickle cells stick together and block blood flow in the body. Mwansa was given a blood b transfusion and medication for her pain that's when Mwansa's mother realized that SCD was a serious condition that can cause health problems. Since then, her parents started following up on hospital appointments. Since then, the treatment of Mwansa hasn't been easy.

How Sickle Cell Disease Affects Mwansa and the Family at Large

Sickle cell disease really affects my niece, so badly. Most of the time Mwansa would have anemia, anemia makes Mwansa pale and tired, and her skin colour turns yellow as well as her eyes and mouth. Sometimes she goes through sudden pain, most often the pain occurs in her chest, arms and legs. She also experiences painful finger and toe swelling, fever fluid loss, pain and a violent cough. Most of the time she goes through blood transfusions, Vaccines, and antibiotics. Sickle cell disease has also affected her education, Mwansa also misses out on some popular childhood activities, like playing games, touch, wider, etc. and sometimes she misses class from time to time or she is absent for doctor visits or hospital days.

Chronic fatigue or pain makes Mwansa less motivated to learn. Sickle cell disease has not only affected Mwansa but her mother and the family at large. It has affected her mother financially, physically, and emotionally. As you know, no mother wants to see their child sick. Most of the time, Mwansa's mother goes through fatigue, stress and has more trouble concentrating and remembering things, it affects her financially in the sense that when Mwansa is sick, her mother's business has to come to stand still, because she has to nurse Mwansa in the hospital. As she is a single parent, Mwansa's father left Mwansa's mother without saying anything and married another woman, and he doesn't even support the child, the reasons why he left known by himself. And as for me being Mwansa's aunty, I try to help with the little I have, as am unemployed. Having said that, Mwansa's mother is so supportive of her child, she loves her so much and takes good care of her. She makes sure she gives her plenty of water to drink 6 to 8 glasses of water a day. This helps prevent and treat pain crises. In some cases, fluid may be needed in a Sickle cell patient. She also makes sure Mwansa is not exposed to high altitudes, cold weather, swimming in cold water, or staying away from sick people and she makes sure Mwansa avoids places or situations with exposure to low oxygen levels, for example, mountain climbing or exercising extremely hard. She makes sure Mwansa eats balanced diet food, and she lets Mwansa participate in physical activities and stay active and rest breaks are advised. Despite all the challenges that Mwansa's mother passes through, she tries her best to live a normal life, and as a family, we try to do a lot of things together. In conclusion, I would like to thank Agnes MN for giving me this opportunity to participate in this book writing and sharing my niece's story.

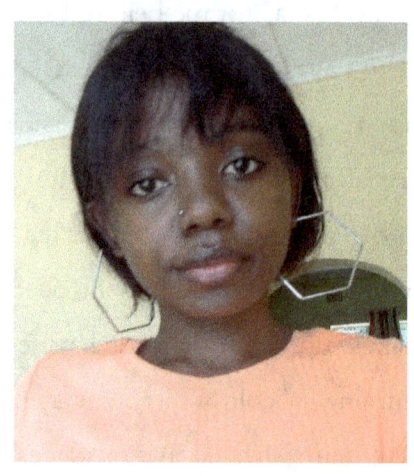

How Sickle Cell Disease Impacted my Family
By Esnart Chushi

My Battle with Sickle Cell Disease (SCD)

It is a severe hereditary form of anaemia in which the haemoglobin distorts the red blood cells in a crescent shape or into a sickle cell shape. The cells die early, leaving a shortage of healthy red blood cells and can block blood flow causing pain, some of the symptoms include anaemia (sickle cells break apart), episodes of pain which is the major symptom of sickle cell anaemia, swelling of hands and feet, frequent infections, delayed growth or puberty, vision problems. Its associated symptoms can have a widespread impact on both the psychological functioning of individual diagnosed and their families. Caregivers are responsible for the physical care and emotional support for those unable to care for themselves. The challenges of caring for a loved one with a chronic disease such as sickle cell disease can be isolating and overwhelming.

My cousin was born with sickle cell disease and my parents took her when she was just a baby because her mom died immediately after giving birth to her due to some complications. No one knew that she had sickle not until 2003 when they noticed that she was not growing fast like the rest of the children that she used to play with. They didn't notice because they had little knowledge about sickle cell disease, they ignored everything thinking that she would eventually catch up with the other kid and she also experienced numerous episodes of pain. She was later on taken to the hospital where she was diagnosed with sickle disease after completing some lab tests but since my parents had little knowledge on how to take care of someone with sickle or even how to manage the disease. It was hard for them, so they started doing some research on how to manage the condition, what to feed them, and what to do when a certain situation occurs. The first few years were a whirlwind-overwhelming and stressful. Because of the frequent episodes of pain also known as crises that she experienced. she was mostly in and out of the hospital, and the episodes of pain that she experienced affected her sleep and she was not able to go to school, not being able to play with us and this made us sad always seeing her sick and unable to play with her. So what we used to do was to sit on a chair with her and just watch TV, we would crack jokes here and there so that she would at least smile and make sure she felt loved by us and so that she knew no matter what, we would always be there for her in whatever situation she was going to find herself in (but before I knew or understood what sickle was, I used to think she used to exaggerated the pain she felt so as for to get all the attention from our parents and we felt neglected by our parents mostly mom because she used to spend most of the time taking care of my cousin which always stopped from working household chores). At some point, she stopped going to the hospital due to financial problems that my parents started experiencing because only my Dad used to work, mom stopped going to the market to take care of the child and because Dad earned little amount and no other family members were willing to help out in supporting her medical expenses or even came to see her despite my mom asking them for help. When she tries to call them on the phone, they ignore her calls. Even her own father abandoned her and disappeared to date, he has never been there for her, and no one even knows his whereabouts. Therefore, the cost of buying medicines, paying for the hospital bills and even transport fare to take her to the hospital became hard for us. Even eating a proper meal became difficult for us.

Things became so bad that we had to go on a break from school for some months until our parents were able to find money to pay our school fees. Dad used to feel bad about not being able to provide for his family and even seeing us all the entire day without going to school used to make him feel sad, at times when his outside seated alone, he would shed some tears and I would go and wipe his tears and tell him not to worry everything will be fine one day and I told him that we understood that it was not his fault that he wasn't able to pay for our school fees because he had important things that he had to take care of. Instead of going to school, I started going to the market to start selling and help with raising some money to take care of my cousin who was sick and to also ensure that my siblings went to school. I continued going to the market and doing some petty work so that I could raise enough money to take home. I knew deep down that my dad felt guilt about everything but he was not able to do anything, and I wasn't willing to just sit down and watch him work himself to death just so he could provide for us and they never gave up they kept on having hope that everything was going to be alright one day.

In 2013, things started getting better so I continued going to school (from 2011 to 2012) and also my siblings and my cousin too started school, she was told and encouraged to participate or engage in school though some kids started mocking her because they said she was too big to be in their class and that she looked unhealthy and called her a sicklier because she would frequently get sick, they also called weak, lazy and that she used to fake her sicknesses just be favoured in a class by the teacher. My cousin never told anyone about what she used to experience in school, she would rather cry alone and even lock herself up in the room and whenever you ask her what's wrong, she would say nothing was wrong but we would actually say that something is indeed wrong because she was a jumpy person and from nowhere, she started locking herself up always because she wanted to be alone and never wanted to go outside to be with her friends or us the family members.

As days went by, her behaviour totally changed, she even told mom that she no longer wanted to go to school just for her to avoid being surrounded by her classmate and mom would accept for her to stay home thinking maybe she wasn't feeling well. My cousin became suicidal and always took the opportunity whenever she was alone to try to kill herself, it was either me or mom who would find her trying to take her own life. She became depressed and thought she was a burden to everyone and felt helpless because of her frequent hospitalization and she wished she had died together with her mother instead of her causing us pain and always making her aunt waste money on her instead of focusing on herself and her family.

One day, mom decided to ask one of her classmates about what was going on with their friend. She was the one who explained everything to mom about how my cousin was being treated by other pupils in class. It was then that she finally understood why she never wanted to go to school, why she became suicidal, and always wanted to be alone. Mom talked to the teachers who later addressed the entire school and told them not to bully their friend's despite of how they look or where they come from because everyone is the same.

Mom went back home and talked to her and told her to open up about such things because it is not easy to deal with these things alone that why she ended up having suicidal thoughts. My parents found someone within the community whom they could talk to (more like a therapist since could not afford a real therapist). As days went by, she started changing and she became the same jumpy person that I had always known but whenever she became quiet, I would cheer her up just to ensure that she did not feel bad. We wrote our grade 9 and we both passed, went to boarding school and this is where things became worse because I was the one who used to take care of her whenever she became sick and each time, she became sick, I would be called out of class to look after her. I couldn't call my parents back home because we were not allowed to go with phones at school and teachers were not allowed to give their phones to students and parents were not allowed to enter school at any time, they would only visit on visitation day. At times, if you took her to the sick bay, they used to think she was pretending to be sick because most people used to fake their illnesses whenever they did not want to attend class or go for prep. Taking care of her in school really affected my grades because I rarely went to classes or even had time to study.

In 2018, a year before we went into grade 12, my cousin became so ill that she started having trouble with walking. At times even talking and would also experience severe headaches. One day, she just became worse and was rushed to the hospital where she died. This was a really sad moment for the family as we had lost someone so dear to us, but I know heaven gained a very beautiful soul and I know you are happy and safe even though I could not believe that you had left me all alone after all the plans that we made about which university to go and we are both going to study. We both decided that we were going to be doctors and try our best to help kids that are going through what she was going through and find ways of educating people on how to take care of their child with sickle disease, but it was sad that we will not be doing the things that we planned together.

In 2019, I wrote my grade exams and I managed to pass. I worked hard for my cousin so that she could be proud of me and so that I could study medicine just as we planned. In 2020 I applied to university after my results came out and I was accepted into university. I'm now a 3rd-year student still working hard so that I finally do what I was born for and so that I can help children out there who are going through what my cousin went through. To date, I still miss her, and I wish she was here with me to support me and just push me to work hard because she is the one who kept me going in high school even when I did not want to study.

Whenever I was nursing her, she would force me to get my books and study, saying being a doctor is not easy and it needs good points for you to be accepted into university. I always cry whenever I miss her, but I know that she is in safe hands, and she is watching over me. I just want to say that I will forever make you proud and despite you not being here, I will still work hard until I become a doctor and save the lives of many people just as you wanted us to do. I will stay focused on my goal until I achieve it no matter what just continue watching over me. All I can say to parents with children leaving with sickle cell is that:

- Never put limits on your children, just let them live their dreams. All they need is your support.
- Educate them so that they can speak up for themselves and become their own advocate.

- Teach your children about their condition.
- Tell them not to feel sorry about their condition. God made them for a specific reason and purpose, their story might encourage someone out there to leave another day.
- Let them surround themselves with people who love them such as family, friends and show support.

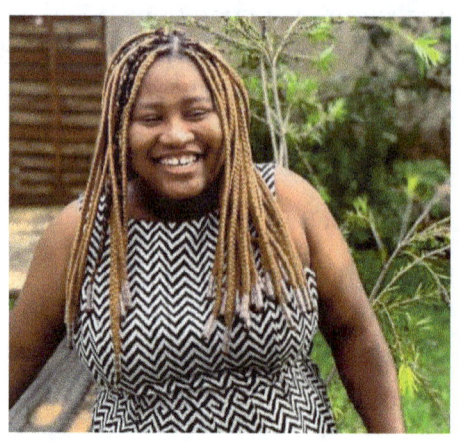

Survival Journey from Sickle Cell
By Esther Ngoma

Introduction

We don't choose which family we are born from or what sickness we are born with, it all happens, and we find it in us or with our friends. Growing up in shanty compounds with no knowledge about sickle cell disease. And our mothers, grandmothers and neighbours have got their own beliefs and cultures to believe in. Without having full knowledge about sickle cell disease, they predicted wrong things about it and they never knew how it comes and what happens next. We believe that when one is born with sickle cell disease, they die before they reach the age of 5. But now we are seeing people grow with it.

Now that our generation knows the threats and the symptoms even how one gets it, gone are those days when people were born and living without the knowledge of sickle cell disease. Seeing your friends, sisters and neighbours dying but you can't do anything, and you don't understand anything of what it is and how it is. The impact of losing someone paying your school fees because of sickle cell, the impact of losing a mother or a brother or a friend because of sickle cell. Am going to share with you the impact it had on my education when my sister I was staying with had a child with sickle cell, and the other impact I had experienced when I went to a boarding school and my roommate had sickle cell.

My School Best Friend Who Lived with Sickle Cell

I went to a boarding school in the East part of Zambia, being far from home wasn't bad. I had a roommate who suffered from sickle cell disease, sometimes she could get sick in class and sometimes skip classes. I wasn't really sure what was wrong with her cause it was my first time seeing someone with sickle cell grow to that age, and for the first time, she told me she lost blood. She was the person I was studying with all the time and doing everything with. Sometimes I would also skip class just to check up on her, how she was feeling at the sick bay. Getting her food and sharing the same room with my sick friend was an experience. Sometimes it would get worse at night and my duty was to call on the house captain and the matron in the teacher's compound.

When it was time to take her to the hospital, I was always there as a friend to help her pack because sometimes she would spend nights in the hospital. I had lost a lot of concentration in school, all I wanted was to rest mostly because my mental health was also at stake, taking care of a friend who is sick was confusing and couldn't get over it at times. Mostly, when she was sick, it was hard for me to study at night and sometimes attend class until the matron picked her up. I took her like a sister and whenever she wasn't fine, I was the first one to know.

Out of ignorance, I would joke around saying let me go and give you blood it seems you are really lacking blood. We used to laugh about it until one day, just after being knocked off from school, she got very sick. I saw her struggling to breathe on the way to the dormitory, so I called for help from the school. I took her to the hospital and that's how I knew that she had sickle cell. I donated my blood for her because my blood group is o positive. Despite receiving blood from a lot of relatives, she still spent about a week in the hospital. That's how I became a blood donor because I saw and understood that our friends in hospitals needed blood.

When we closed school, I thought I would see her the next term, we only heard that she died just after we closed schools. I couldn't concentrate at all, I failed to study alone, and everything took a bad turn for me. I never wanted to go back to school, I felt depressed, studying alone and was worried about how to make new friends again, all this was hard for me. I started skipping class without my parents knowing, due to a lack of concentration, I failed to study for my examinations, and it affected my results. I didn't pass with flying colours like I promised my parents, I gathered my courage and talked to my matron about it, wasn't bad because they had to find someone

I could talk to and help bring my pieces together. She made me meet new people and have friends.

My Sister had a Child with Sickle Cell Disease

Staying with my sister and her husband, a baby born in a family always brings joy but, in this case, it was the opposite. The baby had sickle cell, and the husband left without a word. My sister would go to work and leave the child with me, sometimes the panic of not knowing what to do when she gets sick but only to call her mother from work. After some time, a maid was hired but the maids couldn't stay for long because it was always sickness after sickness, sleepless nights, her food was mostly different, and she was difficult to feed. Maids couldn't take it. Instead, I stayed in to take care of the child knowing very well that there was nothing I could do. Failed to start school because no one will take care of the child, sometimes I used to get upset but since all I wanted was school, I had to keep calm knowing very well that I would start school one day. Knowing very well that it would be okay one day, I stayed without school for a year to 2 years. My friends had passed to other schools and other grades while I was just at home taking care of the child. Sometimes I used to wish there was no sickness in the world because I would have been in school without any obstacles. Sometimes I hated my own life, seeing my friends having fun playing while I was just with the child, I felt bad. When the child was about 3 years, they enrolled her at a private school. I felt l that the day had come for me to proceed with school.

I started telling my friends that I was also starting school, I even had the opportunity to make friends and go play outside. At that time a maid was hired, not bad the maid stayed until I started school, and everything was going swimmingly for me.

At least I was not going to hospitals or clinics or feeding her since the maid was there. My prayer was to finish my school at least. The times we used to spend a week or so in the hospital, I remember seeing her eyes yellow, her mouth and her stomach growing more than usual, it was upsetting to see the toddler using the oxygen machine. Fear gripped my heart. All of this felt like a distant memory to me.

Making her start school was not a bad idea at first because she was growing and meeting new friends; it was amusing for her and everyone else, I suppose. But she still felt sick at times. As for me, going to school was enjoyable and I enjoyed it, even though I was late but thank God I managed. The child had matured to the point where her preferred mode of transportation was running around the home. We had become accustomed to having her around, and we had laughed and played with her, but who knew it wouldn't continue long? She began having breathing difficulties and was rushed to the University Teaching Hospital for medical attention. The first thing was oxygen; people prayed but to no avail; people donated blood but to no effect; only the stomach grew after infusing blood in her. My school was temporarily placed on hold. I had to take care of the house and go by the hospital to take care of her so that her mum could rest. It was difficult for me to focus on everything at school, home, and the hospital. I thought I was too young for all of this. We lost the child in no time, which was unfortunate because I couldn't return to school. Because my sister was depressed and couldn't work or pay my tuition, she couldn't talk to anyone or do anything and preferred to be alone.

We couldn't pay the rent since she had stopped working and I had stopped going to school, so we were evicted from the house. I began moving about with my grandma, asking for assistance. I would move around the neighbourhood looking for meagre jobs to do. At this time in life, I cursed myself because the only thing I ever wanted I couldn't achieve. I thought I'd never be able to return to school because of the grief my sister was through at the time, which affected the entire family. I began working at a bar since no one would assist me with my school tuition. I worked for months, but I was still young for all of it. until we found well-wishers to help me with my school, that's how I stopped working in the bar and had to go to a boarding school and concentrate on school that's how I survived the impact it had on me because who knows, maybe I wouldn't have even gone to school at all if everything had been like that, maybe I would have been in the streets begging until now or doing something else in bars. As for my sister, it was hard for her to survive the pain and everything, she remembered losing her husband just like that and losing the child under her care left her devastated. We lost her after a month; she wasn't sick, but she just fell, then I realised that sickle cell is a bad thing because if not for it, my sister would have been happily married and that child couldn't have died at that age and I couldn't have been missing school or doing meagre jobs just for me to raise money for school. My sister couldn't have died from depression.

The Lesson I have learned.

We believe that sickle cell is inherited from one of the parents. Let's also encourage couples to test if their blood groups are compatible. Because some people lose their marriages, lose their loved ones. And if people test before having kids, it will lessen the disease.

After all these encounters with people who are suffering from sickle cell, have come to learn not to make a joke out of someone's sickness because it seems like an easy thing but what they are going through is not comparable. I used to make jokes with my friend about giving her my blood without the knowledge of how she was feeling deep down in her heart. We should not compare what we go through to what our friends are going through.

I've learnt to care for the people I encounter in my life since I don't know who will save or look after me tomorrow. No one knows what tomorrow may bring, I learnt to gather my self-esteem when trouble arises or am in fear even when things seem to shutter at me. And also I have learnt to share what is troubling me with my close friend. With a disease like sickle cell, let's normalise telling our close friends we are staying with so that when they see a threat it will be easy to control the situation. I will urge every one of us to help our friends and sisters out there who are in need of blood when we know that we are capable of helping. And also, to tell a friend or a stranger about sickle cell disease and save a soul.

Sickle cell disease as a whole I believe it is preventable and that it would have been ideal to test it in the same manner that we test other diseases such as Malaria.

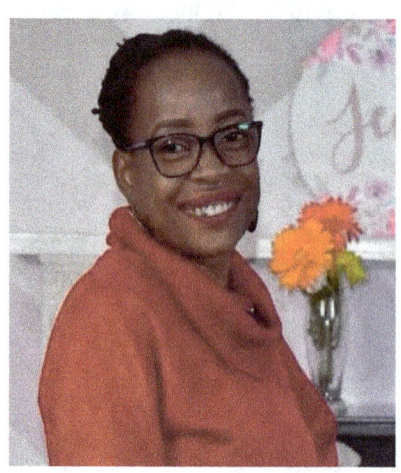

From Patient to Advocate
By Eunice Owino

Today I thank God for turning the pain of sickle cell into my calling and a testimony. I advocate for Sickle Cell Disease to fulfil my God-given purpose on earth. I have done many television interviews talking about sickle cell in three languages (English, Swahili and Luo), Many people do not understand what sickle cell is and why I do what I do. Each and every one of us was born to bring a solution on earth and to fulfil our God-given purpose and call.

"Sickle Cell Warrior" Eunice Owino's Story

Eunice Owino was just eight months old when she developed jaundice, and her parents recognized it with dread as a symptom of sickle cell disease. Another daughter of theirs had died from the condition before Eunice was born.

Now, successful and stronger than ever at 42 years old, Ms. Owino has defied the odds that see more than half of the approximately

1,000 children born with sickle cell disease in Africa every day die before their fifth birthdays – despite the fact that with access to treatment, they can live long and happy lives.

Ms. Owino, who lives in Nairobi, Kenya, has become an advocate – a "sickle cell warrior" – as the founder and leader of Sickle Cell Uhuru Trust, a platform for amplifying the voices of people living with sickle cell disease. In this article, she shares her experience living with sickle cell disease and discusses her work spreading awareness about the condition.

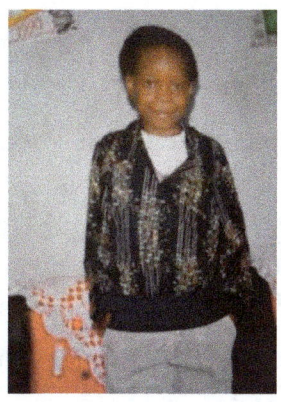

Eunice Owino At Age 9

Growing up, I spent a lot of time in the hospital, especially as a very young child. Those of us with sickle cell disease have to take extra care to stay healthy and avoid sickle cell crises.

Childhood Life

I was diagnosed with Sickle Cell at 8 months old at the Kenyatta National Hospital (KNH). My parents told me that I showed the same symptoms as my late sister, who died before I was born, so when they realized my symptoms, they took me to the hospital, and I got diagnosed with sickle cell disease type SS.

Growing up was very difficult for me because I spent half of my life in and out of the hospital, thank God for the love and care of my family, which helped me to see life in another way. My family treated me as a normal child, nothing different, when I was sick, they were always there for me, and when I was ok, I did house duties as everyone else. I remember the many days and nights I spent in the hospital, including being discharged on 24 December, to have Christmas with family. Sometimes we spent Christmas in the hospital, and that was life growing up.

When I went home, my childhood friends and I used to play all sorts of games, and sometimes I would get crisis at night, which meant that I overplayed and exhausted my body.

One thing I remember strongly was my mum always telling me to put on a sweater, and as I went to the house to pick it up, she would tell me to drink water.

Another thing was always taking these three drugs: folic acid, Proguanil and Ibuprofen throughout, I became so immune to them, that I used to chew them, swollen them and sometimes throw them in the bathroom; but my father would always find them, and would give me a talk, explaining to me why these drugs are very important in my body and my life. As a child, it was very hard to understand, but all in all, we thank God for His wisdom, and I was able to understand myself and take better care of myself.

As I child, I also remember how crises used to come when weather patterns would change from cold season to warm. I would get ill during weather changes or changes in the environment. My grandmother used to give me herbal medicine to inhale, which used to reduce my chest pains. I used to have sensitive skin, but my grandma would apply herbal medicine, and it would clear everything. Those are some of the challenges I went through growing up as a child until I reached 13yrs when I understood sickle cell and I started living a more pain-free life, just doing everything in moderation.

School Life

When I started school, it was very exciting for me. At that time, I didn't really understand what sickle cell was, all I remember is my mum nudging me to drink water, put on my sweater and rest, don't do this or that", don't carry anything heavy. Then when the weather changed from hot to cold and cold to hot seasons, I always used to get sick, and I hated it because that meant that I would have to miss school for weeks or even months.

I am thankful to God for my mum, who was a teacher and used to explain to my class teachers every year as I progressed to the next class about my condition and how they should handle me in times of crisis. I was lucky as the teachers knew me and I was lucky to join Mum's class when I went to class 8. She is the pillar of my strength because she always used to carry me on her back whenever I got sick in school. Also, she was an advocate because she would identify other children with sickle cell disease in our school and would offer support and advice to their parents.

I remember when I was in class 3, I got very ill that year and I think I only attended school for three weeks. Every term, I would only go for the last week when people were doing exams for that year. I can't really explain what was wrong, but all I know is that at that time, I had a very bad crisis because I was given 72 injections all on my behind. I hated anyone wearing white, especially the doctors and nurses, till I became immune to the injections because I was given 3 injections every day. These are what I call dark days in my life, that is when I stayed in hospital for more than two and half months.

When I turned 13 years old, I started understanding my condition, which is Sickle Cell Disease. I tried to be like any normal child by doing extra-curricular activities and also noticed that every time I would enter a swimming pool, I would get a sickle cell crisis and get admitted to the hospital. I would only enter the pool for less than five minutes, and it would cause me to stay away from school for a month or so. I remember also kneeling or any punishment meted out to me, I would go into crisis because of stress, and I would get sick because of that stress.

So, I had to be the best student in all my life so that I don't get punished or get any disciplinary issues in school. I was a very active girl in school, where I was the leader of the Girl Guide in primary and secondary and later on, progressed to be head of rangers; I also got involved in drama and music and we won many trophies during competitions.

In high school, when I got sick, I used to take myself to the hospital and explain to the doctors what was wrong, get medicine and go back to normal life.

College life was nice, and I never had any crises, I enjoyed my studies, where I got a diploma in Community Development, Project Management, Community Health, Social Work, Business Management and Christian Ministry.

I started understanding how Sickle Cell is and how to take care of myself by praying, keeping warm during cold seasons, drinking water (hot, cold or warm), eating vegetables, and fruits, taking my medication at the right time and going for my regular checkups after every three months. This is how I have managed to live with Sickle Cell till today, I live my life as normal as any other person.

Job Life

I started my first work as a sales and marketing executive, then moved to music and entertainment, where I stayed for more than 20 years, then moved to real estate and now am doing advocacy full time.

Life with AVN

I had a very painful hip joint because of Avascular Necrosis which was on and off since 2003. I did my first X-ray in 2005, which showed something like a crack on the hip joint. To reduce or stop the pain, I was put on a lot of painkillers, and none of the doctors told me what it was, only telling me that I needed surgery and at the same time, saying that the surgery is for old people and that I was too young. I looked for a medical explanation until I met a Surgeon in 2013 who explained to me that I have Avascular Necrosis (AVN).

Avascular necrosis (aseptic bone necrosis) of the hip and other major joints may occur as a result of ischemia which is caused by a lack of oxygen in the hip joint called Avascular Necrosis (AVN). He advised that I do the total hip replacement on my left hip or else arthritis would affect the whole leg, which can lead to the leg deforming. Life was very hard, having pain in the hip and it locked at any time and restricted my movements until it turned back to the normal way. It made me miss my job a few times till I was told to get a permanent solution. That's how I ended up doing the hip replacement because now I had knowledge about AVN.

Life After the Total Hip Replacement

After the successful surgery on the hip, I have never had any pain in the hip or fallen down because the hip couldn't stand my weight. I had to rest the leg and maintain joint mobility I used to elevate and rest the joint, physical therapy, and pain relief medicine. I took a month and a half to heal and get back to work, going back to work, I couldn't be my best cause I was on crutches for six months before I could be back on my feet. The surgery was called a total hip replacement.

I have since developed Leg ulcers which occurred at the ankles because of a lack of blood flow and oxygen, it's on both ankles. It is very painful, and it can make you unable to walk for months unless you use crutches to help you move, when it becomes sceptic or inflamed.

A sickle cell crisis is a sharp pain in your joints. When sickle-shaped red blood cells block blood flow, you will feel intense pain where the clog is. Sometimes the pain is so bad it requires a visit to the emergency room. Sickle cell crises are often caused by sickle cell triggers, and everyone has different triggers. The best way to manage sickle cell disease is to know your individual triggers and avoid them. Stress is a big trigger for me (avoid stress or putting myself in stressful situations and I live a day at a time), but other triggers are strenuous exercise or swimming in cold water. The older I became, the more I knew how to manage my condition, and I was not hospitalized so much.

A landmark moment for me as a person living with sickle cell disease was hip replacement surgery. I had been experiencing terrible pain in my hip and would sometimes wake up in the morning, and my hip would lock. After 10 years of pain, finally, an orthopaedic surgeon diagnosed me with Avascular Necrosis (AVN) and recommended hip replacement surgery. AVN occurs when bone tissue dies due to lack of blood supply and is a morbidity of sickle cell disease.

Going through hip replacement surgery was incredibly stressful but worth it in the end. Arranging to pay for the hip replacement surgery through insurance was difficult. If insurance companies know you have sickle cell disease, the hip replacement won't be covered. After the surgery, my doctor explained that I was not healing as well as I should have been because of all the stress, and stress is a trigger of sickle cell. In the end, I made the difficult decision to quit my job and focus on my health. After I healed, I turned my attention to my advocacy work.

Advocacy Work
A Voice for Sickle Cell Warriors

People living with sickle cell disease often refer to themselves as sickle cell warriors. We're called sickle cell warriors because we're fighters. Even though we experience excruciating bouts of pain, we can overcome.

We're called sickle cell warriors because we're fighters. Even though we experience excruciating bouts of pain, we can overcome.

We also have to fight the stigma surrounding the disease, as the biggest challenge of living with sickle cell disease is discrimination. People tend to define me by my condition and characterize me as a hopeless person because of it. Not all doctors have a good understanding of the potential of a person living with sickle cell disease. But because of recent advances in medicine, like treatment with hydroxyurea, bone marrow transplants, and gene therapy, a person living with sickle cell disease can live a long and happy life. That's why I am so passionate about educating people about what's possible for those living with sickle cell disease. There are sickle cell warriors who are over 90 years old!

When I started my advocacy work in rural areas, I met two unrelated children whose parents were told that these children would not survive into adulthood. Neither child had ever set foot in a classroom. They were locked away with the cows because their parents were waiting for them to die and didn't want to "waste" their money on schooling. So many people simply lack knowledge about the condition. Sickle cell disease is not a death sentence. You can live with it and manage it.

Sickle cell disease is not a death sentence. You can live with it and manage it.
I am so motivated to help people understand that children with sickle cell are normal children and need to go to school and clinics. When I came back from this visit, I realized how important it was to share my story and push forward with my advocacy work. When I meet new sickle cell parents in the ward, I hope meeting me gives them hope that their children will live a long life.

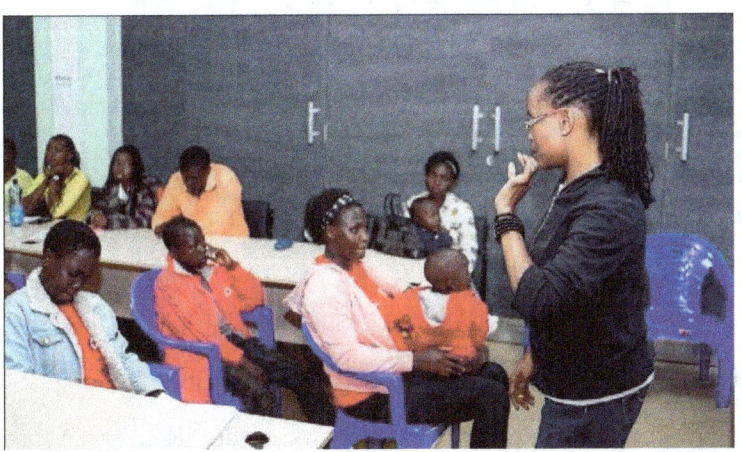

Ms. Owino Working With A Support Group Of Sickle Cell Warriors And Their Caregivers At Moi Teaching And Referral Hospital In Eldoret, Kenya

The best way to eradicate stigma is through education, so my goal as an advocate is to build awareness about sickle cell, especially among healthcare providers in rural areas. My individual advocacy project as a Voices of NCDI Poverty Advocacy Fellow was executed in Homa Bay

County, a rural area of Kenya where I am from and the prevalence of sickle cell is very high. I gave a lecture on what sickle cell is to health care providers and gave tips on how they could explain sickle cell to parents, manage their patients, and administer their medicine. I also led a workshop with patients and parents that emphasized how important it is for sickle cell patients to visit the clinic every month in order to pick up more medicine and have a check-up. This also helps patients build relationships with their doctor so their doctor becomes familiar with the triggers of each patient and the patient has a resource when they're experiencing a crisis.

We also had sickle cell warriors share their experience living with sickle cell disease. This was especially helpful for new sickle cell parents and patients. It is vital to meet members of the community and understand that they have support from others.

Anyone can help by supporting people you meet with sickle cell, especially children. Mental health is so important, and sometimes people living with NCDs need to share their troubles in a space where they feel safe and do not have to worry about stigma from others.

The Future for People Living with Sickle Cell Disease in Africa

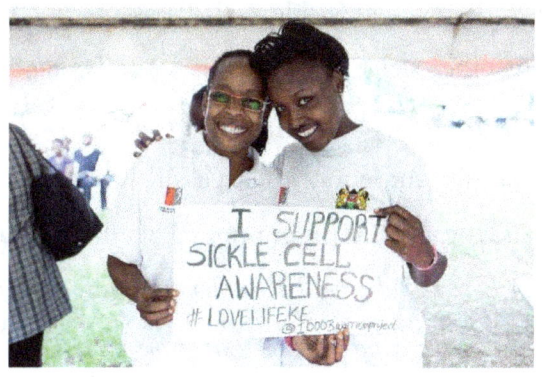

Ms. Owino (Left) Promoting Sickle Cell Awareness On World Blood Donor Day In Nakuru County, Kenya

For years, policy decisions were made that directly affected people living with sickle cell disease and other non-communicable diseases (NCDs), although people living with these conditions were not consulted. I am inspired that people living with NCDs are now sharing their experiences and needs with policy experts, so our voices are heard before these policies are put in place.

The integrated care delivery strategy PEN-Plus is a much-needed solution for the sickle cell disease community, especially on the African continent. PEN-Plus helps people living with sickle cell disease by decentralizing vital diagnosis and treatment services such as hydroxyurea, pain management, education, and counselling to rural areas where the world's most vulnerable people live. Now, people can receive care for sickle cell disease and other NCDs closer to where they live, instead of traveling to the capital city for treatment. I hope all counties in my country, Kenya, adopt PEN-Plus so everyone who needs it has the opportunity to receive chronic NCD care close to home.

I want the world to know that sickle cell disease is not a death sentence and I want other sickle cell warriors to understand that if they take care of themselves, they can live a normal life. We can spread awareness and demand equitable access to healthcare for all through education, advocacy, and programming like PEN-Plus.

The Voices of NCDI Poverty Advocacy Fellowship provides people with lived experience with NCDIs in the countries representing the poorest billion with mentorship, training in building successful advocacy campaigns, financial compensation, and the opportunity to take a voting role in the governance of the NCDI Poverty Network.

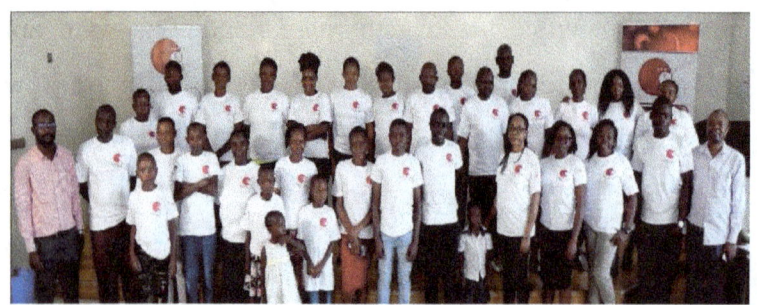

The sickle cell warriors, caregivers and medical personnel in Homa Bay County during the training and

empowering session.

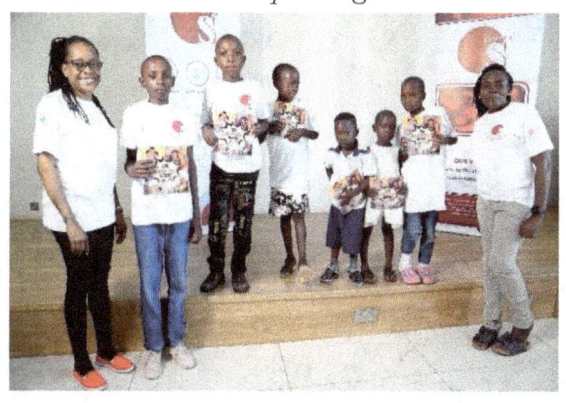

The future of sickle cell in Homa Bay County.

I realized I had a calling to share my story with other warriors who don't have a community to share their stories. Doing advocacy and educating warriors and the whole sickle cell community is what I do every day. God turned my life around when I met him and since then, I have seen life from another angle, he turned my pain into my calling which is helping me to fulfil my purpose on earth.

From my experiences, now am the voice for the Sickle Cell Community in Kenya. I do this throughout the country I haven't reached all the countries affected yet. Just to create awareness, and management for Sickle Cell Patients (Warriors), parents/caregivers. The counties affected are – Nairobi, Kisumu, Siaya, Homa Bay, Migori, Kakamega, Bungoma, Busia, Vihiga, Kisii, Nyamira, Mombasa, Kwale, Kilifi, Lamu, Taita Taveta, Trans Nzoia, Uasin Gishu, Nandi, Nakuru and Tana River.

Ms. Owino is a sickle cell disease advocate and the Founder and Executive Director of the Sickle Cell Uhuru Trust (SCUT), an organization working to create awareness about Sickle Cell Disease, teach about SCD management and emphasises the importance of care for persons living with Sickle Cell Disease in Kenya and around the world.

She is the Regional Coordinator for the African Congress on Sickle Cell Disease (ACSCD), and a member of the Board of Directors of the Sickle Cell Federation of Kenya (SFK). She represents Kenya in the East Africa Sickle Cell Alliance (EASCA), she is an Alumnus of Voices of NCDI Poverty Network, Top 80 most Influencing Sickle Cell Advocate in the world.

She delights in advocating for Persons Living with Sickle Cell Disease and as such, she's represented the plight of SCD patients on various platforms including conferences in Africa and California, documentaries and media interviews across the globe.

Empower a sickle cell warrior, you will empower the whole county. Having sickle cell disease is not a death sentence but a blessing because God knew we could handle it and that's why we are warriors. #liveapurposefullife.

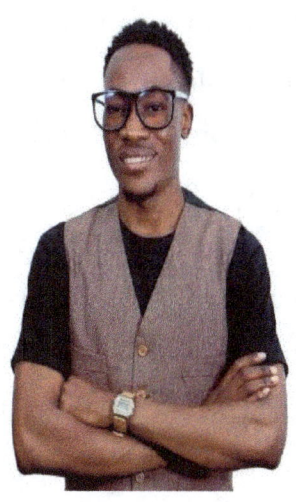

Sickle Cell Warrior
By Ignatius Mulenga Kabwe

About Me

Sixty-kilogram, one point six in height a bit masculine with an interesting posture that's me. Many people tell me there is something about how I stand and walk, perhaps it is because I am from the Copperbelt. Looking back, I was not always like this. I used to be very small, skinny, and always sickly, people often used to wonder and ask me why I had yellow eyes and why I looked pale. However, coming from the place where I come from, all I could say was that I was recovering from an illness.

My name is Ignatius Mulenga Kabwe; I live in Kafue on a farm called Riverside Farm Institute. The farm is in Lusaka province here in Zambia. I am a salesman by profession and a lifestyle coach who specialises in massage therapy and hydrotherapy.

I come from Copperbelt province in a district called Luanshya, township of Mpatatamato. Luanshya was known for copper mining activities back in the day before it was sold. It was in this town where and spent most of my childhood.

I was born in a family of five, my parents and my two siblings. From what I know, my parents were both carriers of sickle cell disease. Unfortunately, I and my two siblings were all born with sickle cell disease. The eldest of us was a girl and the youngest was a boy, I was the middle child.

I have heard people complain about how bad it is to be a middle child, while I do not disagree with them, I cannot complain about it because my experience was not bad at all, being a middle child gave me a chance to have the best of both my siblings.

Growing up, I often hung out with my elder sister, we were so close that when she started her first school, my parent had to enrol me in the same school because I kept crying every time she went to school. One thing about growing up in Luanshya is that; when you are born in Lunshya you are either a child of a miner or a child of a civil servant. Civil servants were more on the educated side than miners, because aside from specialised workers such as operators and managers, most ground wakers were men who were fit and able to work. I was a child of a miner.

Being a child of a miner came with some advantages that others did not have. If you are a child of a miner back then, your father came home every day with bans called Kampompo, these were heavy bans given to miners every day. So, every day, my father came home with

Kampompo and cocoa, sometimes he brought us Thobwa, a powdered instant porridge made from corn. It used to be fun, however, while being a miner's child came with goodies, the downside was that your parents are not as exposed and as informed as teachers and other civil servants.

My parents loved education, although mum was not educated, she was always the forerunner when getting us into school. My father was a technician and I remember wanting to be one after school. Unfortunately, he died while I was still young. My father died after being sick for some time. While it was hard for me and my siblings, it was harder for my mother. She was now a single uneducated woman striving to feed three children with sickle cell disease. To provide for us, she started the business with the little money she got from my father's benefits. While this worked well for us, it actually brought about even more changes in our lives as the nature of her business required her to travel in and out of town more often.

When mum was out, my grandmother took care of us. Not so long after my father died, my young brother fell sick and died from complications caused by sickle cell disease. This was devastating for us and brought even more changes to our family.

My life has been a life of constant changes and accompanied by tragedies. After my young brother died, Mum learned we have sickle cell disease. However, the unfortunate thing was that even though she knew about our condition, she barely had any information about the disease besides what the doctor told her at the clinic. There was no internet for her to educate herself about our condition, which made it even harder for us.

I was 6 years old when I was officially diagnosed with sickle cell disease while hospitalised due to a crisis. I stayed in the hospital for a week. I had been sick often times before being diagnosed and one-time mum had told me that when I was 3 years old, there was a time when I was very sick and I almost died, however, it was not very certain as to whether I had sickle cell or not.

Sickle cell was not very common in my community, not only did this make it unknown, but it also made it hard to talk about it, it was that hidden family secret wasn't supposed to be talked about to our neighbours or even our relatives, mum did not have much knowledge about our condition. One thing I remember from mum is that she was well aware of the fact that we were going to be needing blood every so often. So she always cooked foods that build blood and bought us folic acid to take. Because there was no internet, and no one was talking about sickle cell disease in my community, the only knowledge mum had was the one she got from the clinic, which was not much to help.

she never knew that we needed to keep warm all the time, she never knew that we needed to hydrate all the time, but she knew that we needed blood-making substances and that kind of helped us as much as it could.

When I was discharged from the hospital, I did not know anything about what was happening, however, though I was too young to tell, one thing I knew was that whatever happened was very serious. I stayed away from school for some more time after being discharged from the hospital, and when I went back to school, I could not participate in sports and heavy activities.

Primary School As a Warrior

Being diagnosed with sickle cell disease changed the trajectory of my life at school and at home. My friend could mock me for not participating in school sports and for always being the weak one. They knew I couldn't fight but I was quick to report.

At home, I was this boy who never went out often, nor played sports with friends. This was not because I was aware of the complications of my condition but because my body could not handle most of the activities.

Because I did not go out much, I had a lot of time to draw, play with clay and make cars using wire cars. Making clay pots was my favourite part of being young and probably one thing that I will never stop doing. However, my mother knew that I was not having a balanced life because I was mostly chasing my friends and spending time alone. So, she often chased me out of the house to go and hang out with my friends. I would go and then come back and indoors again. This could go on for some days then again, she would start chasing me again and again.

While I hated going out often with my friends, I think I learned the most valuable lesson in my life and that was the importance of friendship. Back then, I did not know that at some point in my life, friends would be the only people to stand by me as family.

Because Sickle cell disease was not common back home as I mentioned earlier, I never knew anyone who had the condition aside from me. When I was with my friends, I was constantly left out and felt lonely. In primary school, I had a friend, and this guy was my best friend. He was smart and into sports, I often envied him so I could force myself to run, or jump like him.

I remember when I was in grade six, there was a sports competition and I wanted to participate so I signed up for the competition. During practice, as I was running for the first time, I realised why I was told not to run. My heart rate was high, my heart was pounding hard, and I was breathing heavily. Eventually, it was hard for me to breath, and I fell. I do not know for how long I had been down, all I know was that the next thing I saw when I woke up, were my classmates surrounding me and someone shouting, "he is awake, he is awake" When I asked what had happened, I was told I had fainted. When I went home that day, I did not tell mum what happened at school because I knew she was going to shout at me for not listening to her instructions. The next week when I went back to school, I was the kid that fainted. This had hit me hard, and it sent me into more isolation.

Even though no one was talking about me fainting, I became a bit aware of the sigma and the indifference with which I was being treated with.

High School Years.

After writing my grade seven, I went for a holiday. This was my first holiday away from mum. Usually, mum did not like us going on holiday because there would be no one to take care of us. Partly, it was because she did not want people asking about why we often fell sick. But this time, I had managed to convince her that I would be fine and take care of myself.

So I started off from Luanshya to Mufulira for my holiday. Like every young person, I was excited about what would happen on my holiday while waiting for my grade seven results.

When I went to Mufulira, little did I know it would be hard.
For the first time, I was in a house with people who did not know I had sickle cell disease. This was unsettling for me.

When my results came out, I was happy that I had made it to grade eight with good grades and would be in a technical class. This was a class for pupils who performed excellently. Being in the technical class meant I would be taking technical subjects like, technical drawing, woodwork and metal work. Aside from that, it meant I would be in an all-boys class.

In this class, I learned to compare myself to my friends. Being in the boy's class made me realize just how different I was. All my friends were developing and going through puberty at fourteen years old. I saw most of my friends' voices go deep, develop acne, and talk about wet dreams. I was a teenager stuck in the body of a ten-year-old. Getting sick didn't make it any easier, if anything it made me stand out even more, while my grades were not bad, I was the boy who was often sick, often weak, pale, small and couldn't relate to many stories that most teenagers were discussing.

It was during these years of high school that I became conscious of how much sickle cell disease was affecting my life and just how much it was going to affect me. I became more conscience of the complications of my condition and how they affected me.

My academic life slowly changed as I moved from being a pupil to being a student that barely made it on tests.

I remember I was in grade twelve when I first had the first sign of puberty, up until grade twelve, my voice was still sharp, and my face was smooth as always. I remember some girls from my local church called me boy girl because I laughed and talked in the tone of a girl. By this time, I was seventeen years old. At seventeen, all I ever heard was people saying that you have grown when you have your first wet dream. For a seventeen-year-old who had never had one, it always made me wonder.

Because no one knew much about my condition in my area, there was no one I could ask or talk to. I could not talk to mum because she was mostly working, and we just do not have a culture of talking about puberty and sexuality here in Zambia. Girls do get more talks about growing up and womanhood than boys. For boys, you either talk about it with your friends or figure it out on your own.

By this time, I had internet, and I could google a few things about sickle cell disease, unfortunately the internet did not have much data about it as compared to now, I remember the first time I good led the symptoms and complications of sickle cell disease. I was so depressed and couldn't talk about it to anyone.

In my senior year of high school education, I had more fatigue and brain fog and these made school even more difficult, I was going through the first stages of puberty, my body was just starting to change and I did not just have the strength to go through and prepare for exams., I was often down but me and mum had given up going to the hospital because it did not seem as if clinics were helping in any way.

I remember the last time we went to the hospital; I was so in pain with a crisis and they made us wait in a long cue before we could be attended to. It was always like that, long waiting and less attention, no education, and no medication. After waiting for a long cue, we were told to wait for the ambulance so that we could go to the hospital. In the waiting room, I told mum I was tired, and I just wanted to go home because this was not helping at all.

Being at the clinic often meant opening a new file every time you go there, it is still like that in some places. Because some health workers prefer opening a new file for every patient rather than looking for the old files. On the other hand, very, few people are in the habit of keeping their card numbers. So, every time they go to the hospital, they have to open a new file.

For a warrior like me, it meant there was basically no record of my history with sickle cell because we had to buy a new book every time and then get diagnosed for the day.

Some caregivers could see that I had sickle cell disease and write it down, however, most of them could not tell the difference. To them, it was either malaria or some common condition, and because of this, all I received was the care and attention that everyone was getting. Because of these experiences, going to the hospital was just not on the list.

After high school, I stayed at home for some time before I found my first sales job, I still did not know what I was going to study at college but one thing I was sure about was that I needed to do something that was not going to strain my health.

Life after school for me came with even more struggles aside from just crises. I struggled so much with mental health because, after school, everyone was now looking at me as a grown-up. It was then that I realised how hard it was going to be for me as an adult warrior. Because while I was sick, everyone expected me to be like every other grown-up man.

Like in most African countries, men are supposed to be strong, men are supposed to work hard to provide for their families. Men are not supposed to do hard work, play sports, farm and move long distances. Men are not supposed to cry or show weaknesses. Men are not supposed to complain they just take things in and swallow them up. This is the picture of a man commonly known in my country.

The truth is, I am not any of that, I am not strong nor have the strength to do heavy work. The truth is I am sick not like every other male out there. Because of this, I stopped visiting people much or going for holidays because every time I said this work was too hard for me, people just thought I was a spoiled blot that is not going anywhere.

The hardest part of growing up as a warrior has been more than just stigma or the pain and other complications of sickle cell disease. It has been me living under the perception of the ideal man. The kind of man everyone expects me to be.

After working in a boutique for a year, I applied to go to school to study lifestyle coaching, unfortunately, I was rejected because the school had a daily manual work policy, and they thought I was unable to do any manual work. When that failed, I then went on to study marketing and salesmanship, and later changed to lifestyle counselling specializing in massage and hydrotherapy. Over time, I have moved from one practice to another.

Through all these years, I had never experienced better health services as a warrior, there was no one to educate me and my family about possible treatment plans that are available for sickle cell patients, it has always been try and error, moving from one remedy to another and from one herb to another.

Mum was always ready to try out options and medications that she could afford, unfortunately, when I was twenty-two years old. While I was an adult, it was not easy to deal with. I still needed her. Not long after mum's death, my elder sister got malaria and died.

My journey has been a journey of constant change and education, learning how to manage my body with my condition, learning what works and learning how to live with people around me.

With the loss of my family, it is me leaving each day striving to be in better health while in pursuit of meaning.

The death of my elder sister gave me the passion to start advocating for my condition and interacting with other worriers within and outside my country. Advocacy has become one of my passion and purpose. It gave me the dream and desire to seek better health services for warriors in urban and rural places.

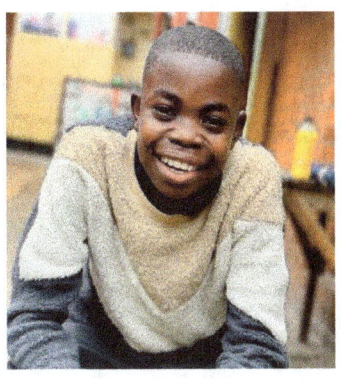

Living with Sickle Cell: A Story of Strength
By Joseph Mubanga

My name is Joseph Mubanga, am 21 years old and I was born on the 22nd September, 2001. I am the second born in a family of 3, two guys and one lady, I live with my mother, my siblings and my 2 nieces. I was diagnosed with sickle cell anaemia when I was 5 months old, so I can safely say am a sickle cell warrior!

My experience being diagnosed with sickle cell has been quite a journey, so I will start:
After 5 months when I was diagnosed with the disease, my mother never believed any of it and what was actually in her mind was, that I had been bewitched, she travelled back and forth to seek pastors for deliverance and suddenly none of it worked. I began to understand my condition at the age of 10 when a doctor at the hospital took time and explained to me about it, since then I would steal my father's phone and research more about it on Google. My condition became a bit intense between the age of 11 and 15 when I was in and out of hospitals and my school became disturbed because

I never learnt a month minus being admitted. I wrote my grade 7 examination with a very swollen face, and I couldn't even move my legs because my joints were hit with a crisis, during my primary school, a few people criticized me about my condition because little did, they understand the condition. I managed to write all the subjects in grade 7 and when the results came out, I had the best results at my school. I continued my grade 8 and 9 at the same school and exactly one week before my grade 9 examination, a crisis hit me this time around I had a very painful one affecting my hands, legs and a very bad toothache! I then was admitted, and all.

I would cry because me and my mother we were 100% convinced that I would miss my exam, but dad tried and convinced the cameraman to come and take a picture of my ID at the hospital and he did, I got my ID card admitted in hospital, during this period, I received blood and some injections for 3 days and I was discharged on Thursday, my exam was starting the following Monday. Monday came and I was still not able to walk, so my father carried me to my class continuously for 1 week and 3 days till I managed to sit for all my subjects, just after my last paper, I was again admitted because I was bleeding from 19:00 to 22:12 continuously when I was taken to the hospital where I was admitted for close to 2 weeks then discharged. The following morning, we received a pastor going around doing evangelism, he shared the Word of God with me and gave me a Bible. Then I received my school results and an acceptance letter to Chilenje South Secondary School. I was really excited because my mind was pretty convinced that I would not make a certificate, but I did, all thanks to the Almighty.

I went to meet the pastor and shared the news with him by then I had met him and shared my story about my condition with him, he then said, pray right now and thank God for this, so we prayed together, and went to the market and got all that was needed to start school. Just after I met the pastor, he would always call me in the morning, afternoon, and night to study the Bible and pray. So that became my habit each day.

On my first day in secondary school, my classmates laughed at me when I entered the class and they shouted, "This is not a grade 1 class, wrong class" because I was very short as opposed to my age, I cried the whole session and went to report to the Head of Departments and they sent teachers to come and tell them about me and my condition and I wasn't ashamed of everyone knowing about my condition because myself already accepted it and moved on. I proceeded with my school but criticism never ended, it grew big and bigger each and every day but I still continued and focused on myself and worried less about my condition, I mastered my morning routine which is "wake up, read one verse of the Bible, pray, take a folic acid and off I go" at this stage now, I decided to put myself in charge of my health and school, I would always check my appointment card with the hospital and go for reviews myself on the appointed date no mess up. In 2017, when I was in grade 10, in my second term, my father passed on just after a short illness and we travelled from Lusaka to Kitwe, where the funeral was being held, I learned from

January to April without a crisis, we attended the funeral and came back in May without a crisis. Now just after we came back, my mother had high blood pressure and was advised by the doctors to stop overworking that she might encounter a stroke, so I and my elder sister decided that she stop working and that me and my sister would provide rent, groceries and other utility bills, so she stopped working I then called the pastor to say I need a part-time job from 06:00 to

12:00 and went to school and applied that I would be changed from morning classes to afternoon classes so that I could accommodate the part-time job. So, I worked at an internet café from 06:00 to 12:00 then went home and prepared by 13:00 am in class. My sister got a job as well as a maid because she never finished grade 12, she went up to grade 9 only. We supported the family we were only 4, my mother, my elder sister, me and my young brother. Just after 3 months of my sister working, she stopped and found a job at a nightclub and ran away from home, we tried but couldn't find her, just there and then I noticed that it was me or no one, I continued supporting my family alone hardly experiencing any crisis. During this period, I never had any savings because my responsibility became very intense and all my salary went towards rent, groceries and other bills, I couldn't buy clothes or shoes for myself or even save a little no.

I continued my school with my side job up until I did my grade 11 to grade 12, then in the midst of my third term in grade 12, a crisis struck again after a long time, I struggled with it for more than a month, I missed 2 subjects and only managed to write 6 subjects on my final exam, at that point, I felt like giving up, I felt very sad knowing I won't make a certificate, either way, I must continue because everyone looking up to me. I could tell that all this pressure was leading me to a crisis, but I must do it because no one else would provide apart from me, after I got discharged, I continued working full time till now.

Because I got to work more to earn more, I experienced a crisis from time to time because of overworking, I continued with my timely hospital reviews and continued working.

During this journey, my mother carried a number of myths about sickle cell anaemia.

- Sickle cell patients do not exceed 21 years old.
- Sickle cell patients cannot marry or get married.
- Sickle cell patients cannot have children.
- And many more..

Along this journey, she was 100% convinced that each day would be my last, and in her everyday prayers, you hear her saying "let all those that bewitched him be judged accordingly" It got more and more uncomfortable when you heard her tell myths to her friends.

This whole experience got me to know more about myself and my condition, it gave me the zeal to be more than what is expected from me and to even research more.

During my work time after grade 12, I never had the privilege to do tours and errands because my boss also was convinced that this disease could strike anytime any minute, so I spent most of my time at the café doing walk-ins and spending my free time on research. My workmates thought I was treated better than all others because my boss would make sure I ate early in the morning before I stated any work, he would ensure I ate lunch on time and kept warm when it was cold. He'd give me holidays during the week, none of my workmates wanted me near them, and they all treated me as if I was working against them.

My only aim was to outperform, deliver and ensure I got my fair share from the company.

In 2020, after a crisis, I was admitted to the University Teaching Hospital and the doctors recommended that I go for an operation because something was growing in my stomach, and I needed to get it removed because it was growing bigger. First, I was sent for an x-ray and given a date to go and do another x-ray, then an operation. After the first x-ray, I went home I was so scared of an operation, so I called my pastor and explained that to him, he just told me to pray. I sat home every day looking at it and praying about it, the next x-ray was after 2 weeks that time came, and we went back for the second x-ray, and I was told that it was smaller than the first x-ray, I was very happy that I won't undergo an operation. And on the last x-ray, it was completely gone.

It gave me more hope to say the condition is not the end of things but rather, the starting of a testimony. It was the beginning of a new chapter, I believed to say God would make an example of me and I was convinced to say a huge testimony would surely come from me and my testimony would run throughout the world.

In 2020, while I was still working, I registered my name "JOSETECH BUSINESS SERVICES" with Patents and Companies Registration Authority, I started providing other services in the Internet café that were not offered, by then my main aim was to actually earn more than I used to earn so that I can continue to sponsor and support my family, I started offering computer lessons in the same space as well, after my employer saw that it was beneficial, he offered me to continue using his space for my services on a certain percentage, I agreed to it and we signed an agreement. I made quite more than I used to earn and bought myself a laptop. In just a few months, I bought myself a printer machine because now my plan was to go and be independent in my own rented shop. Before I could move, the business of my employer started to collapse because limited services were offered there and no proper accounting of money was done, he used to get all the money we made every day and use it, but he failed to pay all of us and some employees left.

As time went by, his business was completely shut down. So, I asked to rent the shop which was once an internet café and continued offering the same services and even more services though with limited equipment, by then with only one laptop and one printer, either way, I carried out my services diligently with passion and transparency and I continued researching and adding some more services to my business catalogue.

In early 2021, I had another crisis that affected my legs, and I was admitted for 2 weeks, when I was discharged, I couldn't even walk, I started learning how to walk from scratch like a baby. My business was completely closed during this whole period, I stayed home for 1 whole month just doing exercises and practicing how to walk again and it took quite some time. My mother decided that we go to the village and seek help because it was worse this time around, I refused to go, but after a month, I started walking and went back to work. Within one month of resuming my business, my pastor who was my former employer passed on and the entire building was closed. We went through till his burial, just after his burial, I was told I couldn't continue using the office anymore because it was meant for administration purposes only by his children. I then went and looked for a job at a shoe store where I worked for a month because the owner said I am not suitable for the job because he wanted me to work 7 days a week without going to church so I stopped. I then looked for another job at a phone shop where I did repair software for smartphones, I worked there for 2 weeks when my former employer's children called me and told me that I could operate from their office provided. I worked for them to collect rentals on their behalf monthly, that's when I went back and resumed my usual business, and I occupied the office space free.

So, life living with sickle cell requires and educates you to endure, to be persistent and to conquer, it requires a steadfast conscious. Most of the time, these things always come in the same package; once you realize you have it, your adventure begins, and those traits begin to work. Have seen cases where people go to seek healing from witch doctors who completely believe that you have not exercised your endurance, quite right at some point, the pain can be unbearable but always remember the Lord has a plan already outlined for a testimony to come through you. I have seen some cases where warriors will only come to the hospital when it's very bad, but the package comes and requires you to be persistent and ensure that you check in and see how you are moving health-wise. I have as well seen cases where warriors sit and can't do anything simply because they are told and their mind is convinced that am sick hence the package comes with the energy to conquer and be whoever you want to and run whichever company you feel like, to pursue and conquer what you are good at beautify your skill and be better at it. You are built with a steadfast conscious to decide and approve which decision based on your benefit health-wise, the conscious will tell you that this is bad for your health, and this is not, do not engage in harmful situations and abuse that consciousness.

During this whole experience, not all my family members understood it at some point, they even thought I was pretending including my own siblings because they had little information about the condition, the reason I did research about it because no one was willing and interested to hear about it anymore. So, from the start, it's been always me or no one. They might be someone committed and be there for you but again, you must have self-interest to just go for it.

My business was completely built based on determination and the passion to conquer and have my fair share of the world in business, it was built on strict modification from my comfort and conviction that I had sickle cell to extremes where I discovered and beatified what am good at in a vast period. During my business adventure and through my own research interest and determination, I have managed to get 2 more computers, 2 multi-purpose printer machines and a very reasonable and clean office space, I managed to provide for my family without fail.

As of now, Josetech Business Services has registered more than 80 companies and business ventures, it has registered more than 10 co-operatives, it helps more than 80 companies be compliant and as well, provides tax solutions, it has provided a number of software solutions for smartphone users and computer users, and it has provided diligent office solutions and stationery. It is a one-stop shop for all your graphic and printed designs.

My plan for the near future is firstly to retake my failed subjects and rewrite them so that I apply to study ICT Software and Hardware, I want to open a repair shop where I can offer software and hardware repairs for smartphones and computers.

Josetech's vision is to be the leader in terms of providing the best products and services as well as professional secretarial and office solutions. By January 2023, Josetech Business Services will have 2 branches including a mobile kiosk that will provide e-government services as well as e-payments. By mid-2024, it will have at least 4 branches empowering about 8 youths. One of these will be the main branch which will provide various services including a computer educative centre and a tuition centre, at least 50% of the total people running this centre will be sickle cell warriors to help them be active and master as well as beautify their skills.

Lastly, I would like to encourage each and every warrior out there that sickle cell is not a curse nor a bewitched sickness rather it's a condition that will make you not different from others but rather better and smarter than others, it's a condition which comes with a huge expectation but again, with the tools to help quench it, of course, it will fight you but you must fight back because you are more than a fighter rather a conqueror, we are born to conquer and achieve mighty than others, we must not compare ourselves with other because in us is a fierce motivation and anger to craving to achieve, all in all, the Lord remains Mighty and Able to do that which is Just!

Regards,
Joseph Mubanga.

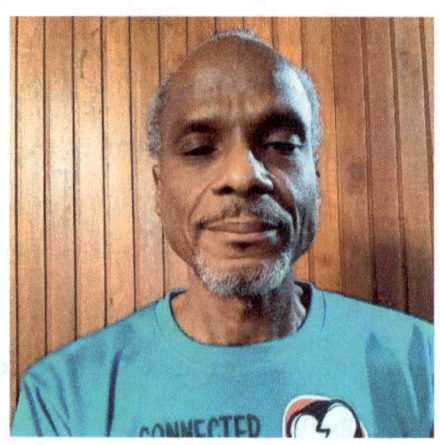

My Sickle Cell Challenges Journey
By K W Young

The journey of 1000 miles begins with a single step, my journey with Sickle Cell SC began 61 years 10 months to date with a crawl. It forces you to pay attention & *"Every decade my body response living with this condition changes"*

0-09yrs found me, Skinny, Not liking to eat, falling asleep at the meal table and having Water Bladders. Crises were frequent and health in retrospect was on a limb. I, for example, loved and still do the beach however the beach/salt water didn't like me due to **(OSMOSIS)**

There isn't much recollection of these years save for pain and protection as my parents figured things out. Staying alive was the goal, I guess, so NO camping allowed e.g.: Boy Scouts & only little beach going.

10-19yrs Diagnosed at 9 years with SC after 2 failed attempts (as told by parents). They were told the magical words, Nutrition / Nutrition / Nutrition by Dr. Harold Nunes, who remained my GP till my late twenties. Nutrition was taken with folic acid (still take it daily). Pain meds included Beserol & Panadol. Test certificates helped to speed up treatment often as nurses/doctors had limited knowledge.

Diagnosed with Meningitis at 12 years old, this became a pivot in care as death came calling. The experience had me• Hallucinating BADLY • MAJOR headaches • spent Weeks in hospital • Couldn't walk for weeks after discharge • breathless having a Bathing. This is where keeping the condition private began I think: Once it was shared with a group leader & their recall *'was, I had*

'Leukaemia and couldn't lift a table.'

During this time, I passed the common entrance (entry to secondary school) and ventured to a cold space. That lasted for 3yrs till transfer to a school closer home was done. I graduated from school with 1 subject (5 was full certificate). Then studied privately plus did woodwork & sign painting. Nonetheless, I had a very active physical life with Tobago vacations, hiking, liming, youth groups, etc. (learning service & leadership)

My Parents played significant roles both focused on aggressive nutrition. Individually, my father created an independent space/mindset & Mom was protective and weary of what the future held/holds (at 94 years she still has concerns, dad passed on, on 1 Sept 2012). I CARE gave her Sickle Cell, genotype. AS **20-29** this is when ASTOR was found & I met FLOWERs, 2 significant LIFE persons to this day, DANCE & HEART. Outdoor life was intense from spending nights on the beach, hiking extensively (did 940 meters), having my son (thanks to his mom), did tertiary technical education in visual design formally & Audio Visual/Video tech informally. This journey was intense learning & doing things I'm gifted with, so often I worked for free & got paid eventually.

SC kept popping up, of course, one Champagne sip created a hospital stay with ACS (acute chest syndrome) and a Blood Transfusion by Dr. Waveney Patricia Charles for a couple days one time.

She was again found via a conference that led to my entry to specialised care at a Haematology clinic where she led many sickle cell lessons. The types of medicines started to change here.

30-39 Began work at CAREC in 1990 & travelled somewhat. Met JC who guided me through the company & remains a friend today. While on DUTY travel (working in another island or country) one year I had a major crisis. I was taken care of by Chryss mainly & co-workers. Chryss helped to save my life & has also filled gaps of 2 days in my memory of that experience. I believe that was amnesia. All the while I never mentioned my condition and doctors wouldn't tell chryss due to confidentiality, I'll always be grateful to her for care giving unconditionally. The lesson here is to speak up. She said, *if you don't want people to know your business don't invite them to your illness* (paraphrase) While hospitalised another time with no relief, I had two major lessons. Jovonne asked, *"did you tell the Drs what your resting HB is?"* I had no clue what that meant. She chided me and gave me time to get the info before she called back, I reported on the call back.

After complaining that this recovery is taking too long, Janelle asked *'don't you know that you body won't use 0.9 saline as well when you get older?'* Tell Drs to try 0.5 of lactate ringers, no clue again. Told the consultant about the saline he didn't listen. Junior Dr. came, told him he tried it, and in less than 24 hrs I self-discharged. These 2 women remain in my life, and I always remember their significance. The body's response to treatment was significant. Emotionally, it taught me the benefit of having someone with the disorder in your life, as lived experiences can save lives.

Studied in Europe twice, in 1992 & 1995, both in Dutch winter. I did dance classes, twice a day 4 days a week. Here, I had another major crisis & walked myself to the hospital in the dead of winter alone and took the bus back. It was a great hospital A&E (accident and emergency) experience. The lessons learnt served me well as I knew the treatment regime & the team followed the letter.

Met Toung on this trip, we became very close when I volunteered to support her through illness and early departure to home for treatment. Initiation into care giving began then with me knowing it. We remain friends today.

40-49 after spending 2-3 full crisis days in the hospital, a caring nurse said, "Sir you can try these", Ibrupofen 1200 (I think). Knowing this dose was many times the normal I held on to it for hours till the body said, ***"just USE the d...... thing"***. I took it, awoke sweating and in absolutely no pain. My bed neighbour said it was the best he had seen me during the stay. Can't recall 24hrs at least of that stay (my son filled me in), another bout of amnesia? I self-discharged 1 day later. Used a cocktail of pain & supplement intervention function 3hrs after getting home to fulfil a promise made before being warded of Power washing the yard & delivering lunches that day. The expectation to perform as usual was rejected by me as I knew the cocktail was at work & any stress would cause a relapse, worse than before.

Earlier submission to emotion & connection led to 6yrs in the USA on marriage *holiday & a Triangle love with Flowers*. I was taught & practiced Interdependence with the significant implementation of that learning today. Self-care was at the core having a 1-week hospital experience during this time though I walked in wintertime to work. Joining the Sydenham Clinic Health System gave me great support, assisted me in getting health insurance, introduced me to the flu shot (which I didn't take), advised me of how AVN worked and precautions to take, and taught me about infarcts and long-term effects. Navigation of the health system was given for Surgery for Eyes & Hernia.

These changes occurred at this time:
Get in front of Pain very early or go for institutional treatment aggressive responses to hunger.
Refocused on Nutrition- food & supplements (health over clothes) Better understanding of and being very comfortable with me & change.
The blessing of my 1st grand child plus the discovery of latent Belief & Strength.
50-59 at Haematology clinic Curtis & Luanne cordoned me off with IBD (inherited blood disorder) information that led me in 2014 to 'Found tribe support in SISBD' and met Dr. Charles' passion in her community here. Here I Spoke up/out differently, it was about sickle cell, and I didn't before.

That quickly transitioned to, supporting others with IBDs & Community Project evolution.

Personally, I had more Eye issues i.e.: bleeding, and soft vision (retina pull) plus discovered Meningitis causes hearing issues & is common in sickle cell disorder. I was no more in the dark about how.

Change happened where the last sentence ended, I Joined Dretchi (hearing support clinic) after some years of treatment, I began hearing better. The doctor said that's not common. This allowed a *change in the way things are seen so things seen changed* e.g.: the benefits of SC. These now are some thoughts, Pain tells a story, Nutrition before medications, the Covid can help teach & Non-conditional Patients with patience. Here are new ways I describe Sickle Cell Life:

- Service For Treatment Client for Patient
- Discomfort for Pain
- Person with SCD Or Warrior for Sickler Connector Or Ambassador for Advocate Earning My Lived PhD For Problems

During this time & because of action in the tribe, more rural I became a mentee to Mr. Edlyn Esdaile & subsequently Mr. Mervyn Virgil. These two men take caregiving very intensely and are as visible as the mothers in care, more visible in the community. Submitting to this guide more of Mr. Esdaile these experiences evolved: 5 Care Pillars mindset, learning by immersion, condition modification: hydroxyurea, met Tamika Moseley (she's a cornerstone of nutrition benefit), use of the principle: be / do / have, community focus, gave/shared widely because I can & attract global tribe with African base.

60-61 &now early 2022, I engaged in 'big people ting' (had been a while) & *a crisis followed pleasure o*f course it's worth it, ALWAYS IS. The thing is I know/knew what triggered it:
- Little water
- No sleep
- Hunger

I knew and tried to get IN FRONT of the discomfort (not word pain) Service was sought at a Health Centre, but the doctor decided not to see me per protocol. Went to the A&E after contacting support from 2 institutions, support was offered at one **that contact was a divine moment.**

That experience came after a broken right foot in 2021, the cause has led to investigating bone
Lesions todecide   ifAVN, myeloma   or   something else.
            In   the meantime,   I
walk/eat/supplement to support my bones. My Learning continues. The change this decade begins with crisis response, my Body pulsates even at rest, Posture to relieve pain didn't work or as well. Consuming animal protein keeps the four responses to hunger at bay.

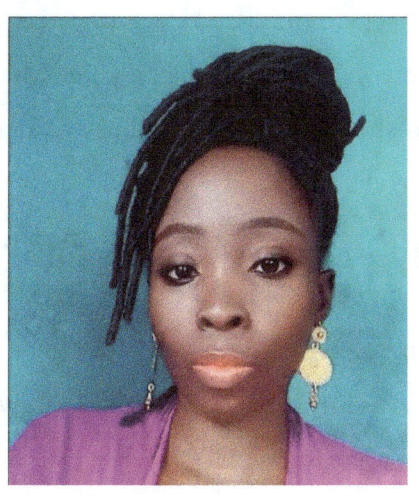

Igniting Hope: My Journey with Sickle Cell and the Fight for Better Healthcare in Nigeria"
By Oluwakemi Oguntimehin

Introduction

In Nigeria, sickle cell disease is a prevalent condition that affects millions of people, including children and adults. This inherited blood disorder is caused by a genetic mutation that affects the structure and function of hemoglobin; the protein responsible for carrying oxygen throughout the body. Sickle cell disease causes a wide range of symptoms and complications that can significantly impact a person's quality of life and shorten their lifespan.

As someone who has lived with sickle cell disease my entire life, I have experienced firsthand, the challenges and struggles that come with this condition. From excruciating pain episodes to hospitalizations and limited physical abilities, sickle cell disease has affected every aspect of my life. However, I have also learned to persevere and overcome these challenges, and I believe that sharing my story can help shed light on the realities of sickle cell disease in Nigeria and inspire change.

The Twist of My Sickle Cell Diagnosis

They say that ignorance is bliss, but for me, it was a prison. A prison that kept me in chains of pain, fear, and misunderstanding for far too long. It all started when I was a young child, growing up in a small town in Nigeria. I was always sick - suffering from stomach aches, constipation, anemia which made me receive countless blood transfusions and various complications that left me feeling weak and exhausted.

My parents took me to the hospital, but the doctors couldn't seem to figure out what was wrong. They ran tests and prescribed medication, but nothing seemed to help. My parents were at a loss, and I was left to suffer in silence.

One day, my parents decided to have me tested for sickle cell, a genetic blood disorder that affects millions of people worldwide. The results came back negative, indicating that I did not have sickle cell. My parents breathed a sigh of relief, and we all moved on with our lives.

But my body told a different story. As I grew older, my symptoms became more severe. I missed school frequently, and my classmates began to call me "Sickler." As I grew older, the stigma surrounding my condition became unbearable. My peers in school labelled me a "sickler," mocking me and shunning me from their circles. At home, my parents' religious beliefs led to accusations of witchcraft and unnecessary exorcisms. My health continued to deteriorate, and I found myself facing multiple blood transfusions, constipation, fatigue, osteomyelitis, and a host of other complications.

I saw a Dr wrote Sickler on my card, I was curious. I asked my parents about it, but they brushed it off, telling me not to worry, that it was because of my frequent sickness that made him write Sickler.

As I entered my teenage years, the stigma surrounding sickle cell became even more apparent. People would look at me with pity or disgust as if I had brought this condition upon myself. I felt isolated and alone, struggling to keep up with my coursework and social life while dealing with the constant pain and fatigue that came with sickle cell.

It wasn't until I was 18 years old and enrolled in university to study biochemistry that I started to believe I lived with sickle cell. Despite this, my parents didn't want to accept. I was struggling to keep up with my classes, constantly battling exhaustion and pain. I couldn't keep up with the classes and I was getting sicker.

There, I experienced splenic sequestration - a condition where the spleen becomes enlarged and traps red blood cells, causing a sudden drop in haemoglobin levels. I needed six blood transfusions to recover, and it was at this moment that I was officially diagnosed with sickle cell disease.

The relief that washed over me was indescribable. For years, I had been labelled a "Sickler" and accused of being possessed by demons, when all I needed was proper medical care and a diagnosis. Finally, I could put a name to my pain and start to understand how to manage it.

Looking back, I can't help but wonder how different my life might have been if I had been properly diagnosed earlier. The stigma and misunderstanding surrounding sickle cell had made my journey all the more difficult, but it had also made me stronger and more determined to help others who are going through similar struggles.

Now, as a biochemist and advocate for sickle cell, I am committed to spreading the word about this condition and the importance of early diagnosis and proper care. The journey with sickle cell is not an easy one, but with the right resources, support, and mindset, it is possible to live a full and fulfilling life.

As I reflect on my journey, I'm reminded of the countless other children who are currently living with sickle cell disease in rural communities across Nigeria. For them, the challenges are even greater, as they often lack access to proper healthcare and are stigmatized by traditional beliefs that label them as outcasts and witches.

It is for these children that I launched the Ignite Sickle Cell Initiative, an advocacy organization aimed at providing support, education, and resources to those living with sickle cell disease in rural communities. Through this initiative, we've been able to provide free routine medications and access to proper healthcare for children living with sickle cell disease. We've also worked to combat the stigma and misconceptions surrounding the disease, providing education and resources to both parents and healthcare providers.

But most importantly, we've been able to give these children a sense of hope and dignity. For too long, they have been neglected and marginalized, left to suffer in silence due to the ignorance and superstition of those around them. But with our help, they are finally able to live a life of dignity, free from the pain and suffering that has plagued them for so long.

As I continue to work towards my goal of ensuring that every child living with sickle cell disease has access to proper healthcare and support, I am constantly reminded of the importance of my mission. Through my work with Ignite Sickle Cell Initiative, I am able to give these children a voice, a sense of hope, and a brighter future.

And so I press on, fuelled by the knowledge that my efforts are making a difference in the lives of others. For me, there is no greater purpose than this - to give hope to those who have been left behind, to fight for those who have been marginalized and stigmatized, and to ensure that every child living with sickle cell disease is able to live a life of dignity and fulfilment.

Purpose of Writing this.

As someone who has lived with sickle cell disease in Nigeria, I know firsthand the struggles and challenges that people with this disease face every day. My own journey has been one of pain, uncertainty, and stigma, but also one of resilience, determination, and hope.

Through sharing my story, I hope to raise awareness about the urgent need for better healthcare, support, and understanding for people with sickle cell in Nigeria. My experiences illustrate the devastating impact of this disease on individuals and families, and the urgent need for action to improve the lives of those affected.

I believe that my story has the power to inspire change, not just in Nigeria but around the world. It is a call to action for leaders, policymakers, and healthcare professionals to prioritize sickle cell disease and invest in the resources, education, and research needed to combat this disease and support those living with it.

I am committed to using my voice and my platform to advocate for change, to break down the barriers that prevent people with sickle cell from living full and healthy lives, and to ensure that every child with sickle cell in Nigeria has access to the care and support they need to thrive.

I believe that together, we can create a world where sickle cell disease is no longer a source of pain and suffering, but a condition that is understood, treated and ultimately cured. And I am proud to be a part of that movement for change.

Sickle Cell in Urban Area in Nigeria

In Nigeria, sickle cell disease is a prevalent condition that affects millions of people, including children and adults. It is estimated that over 150,000 new birth occurs yearly and over 5 million people in Nigeria are currently living with sickle cell. It is estimated that only 75% of these newborns will see their fifth birthday making sickle cell a silent killer of children in Nigeria.

This inherited blood disorder is caused by a genetic mutation that affects the structure and function of hemoglobin, the protein responsible for carrying oxygen throughout the body. Sickle cell disease causes a wide range of symptoms and complications that can significantly impact a person's quality of life and shorten their lifespan.

As someone who has lived with sickle cell disease my entire life, I have experienced firsthand the challenges and struggles that come with this condition. From excruciating pain episodes to hospitalizations and limited physical abilities, sickle cell disease has affected every aspect of my life.

Living with sickle cell disease in Nigeria's urban communities is a difficult journey. While urban areas are home to some of the country's best medical facilities and resources, the challenges faced by people with sickle cell disease are still significant. We will explore the unique challenges and experiences of living with sickle cell disease in urban Nigeria.

Challenges Faced by People Living with Sickle Cell in Urban Areas

Urban areas in Nigeria can be bustling with activity, but they also come with their own set of challenges for people living with sickle cell disease.

High Cost Of Medical Care:

This is one of the major challenges of many people with sickle cell disease. Many struggle to afford the cost of regular check-ups, medications, and hospital visits. Even with medical insurance, the out-of-pocket expenses can quickly add up, leaving many patients struggling to make ends meet.

Lack Of Awareness And Understanding Of Sickle Cell Disease Among The General

Population: This can lead to discrimination and stigmatization, making it difficult for people with sickle cell disease to receive the support and care they need. Discrimination in the workplace, in schools, and in social settings can all have a negative impact on the mental health and well-being of people with sickle cell disease. Despite efforts to raise awareness about the condition, many people still believe in harmful myths and stereotypes about sickle cell disease. Patients may be ostracized or treated unfairly by their communities, and even by healthcare providers who may not understand the nature of their condition despite the low awareness, it is far better than those in rural communities.

Benefits of Living in an Urban Area if You Live with Sickle Cell
Medical Facilities and Resources Available:

Despite the challenges faced by people with sickle cell disease in urban areas, there are some medical facilities and resources available that can make a difference. In Nigeria's major cities, there are specialized sickle cell clinics and hospitals that provide comprehensive care for patients with sickle cell disease. These facilities offer a range of services, from routine check-ups to emergency care, blood transfusions, and pain management. Access to professionals in sickle cell management is also a plus.

Coping Mechanisms and Support Groups:

In addition to medical facilities, there are also support groups and advocacy organizations that provide much-needed resources and assistance to people with sickle cell disease. These groups offer emotional support, education, and information about available resources, as well as advocacy efforts to improve the lives of people with sickle cell disease.

Living with sickle cell disease in an urban environment can be overwhelming, but there are coping mechanisms and support groups available that can make a difference. Many people with sickle cell disease find comfort in connecting with others who share their experiences. Support groups provide a safe space for people with sickle cell disease to share their struggles, ask for advice, and receive emotional support.

There are also coping mechanisms that can help people with sickle cell disease manage their symptoms and improve their quality of life. These include lifestyle changes such as staying hydrated, avoiding extreme temperatures, and getting enough rest. Regular exercise, stress management techniques such as meditation and deep breathing, and seeking counseling or therapy can also be helpful. All this can be easily accessed when in an urban area.

In conclusion, living with sickle cell disease in Nigeria's urban communities can be a challenging experience, but there are resources and support available that can make a difference. From specialized medical facilities to support groups and advocacy organizations, there are many ways to find the help and support you need. By taking advantage of these resources, connecting with others who share your experiences, and finding effective coping mechanisms, it is possible to manage the challenges of sickle cell disease and live a full and meaningful life.

Sickle Cell in Rural Communities in Nigeria

I sat in the back of the jeep, jostled around by the bumpy dirt road as we made our way towards a small village Iboropa Akoko a rural area in Ondo state Nigeria as we were heading there for a medical outreach and the driver, a local from the nearby town, had agreed to take me there to meet with families affected by sickle cell disease. As we neared the village, I couldn't help but feel a sense of dread because as someone who grew up in rural communities and had my own fear share of difficulty and misunderstanding, I knew that the challenges faced by people living with sickle cell in rural communities were often even more daunting than those in urban areas. And this is why the work we do in Ignite Sickle Cell Initiative is such an important one that is renewing hope for both caregivers and their children living with sickle cell.

Challenges Faced by People Living with Sickle Cell in Rural Areas

The challenges faced by people living with sickle cell in rural areas were numerous and often overwhelming. For one, medical facilities and resources were often scarce, making it difficult for people to receive the care and treatment they needed. Many villages lacked even basic healthcare facilities, and those that did have them were often understaffed and under-resourced. And even a lot of people living with sickle had been turned down at many primary healthcare facilities due to not knowing what to do to help them, especially during the sickle cell crisis. This meant that people with sickle cell disease often had to travel long distances to access the medical care they needed, which could be prohibitively expensive, time-consuming and difficult, especially with fewer vehicles on the road and bad roads leading to many of these communities.

Lack of Medical Facilities and Resources

The lack of medical facilities and resources in rural areas was a major barrier to effective sickle cell care. In many villages, there were no hospitals or clinics, and even if there were, they often lacked the necessary equipment, medications, and trained medical personnel to properly diagnose and treat sickle cell disease. This meant that people with sickle cell disease often went undiagnosed or received substandard care, which could lead to serious complications and even death. As a result, many people living with sickle cell disease in these areas are forced to rely on traditional and often harmful practices for treatment.

Lack of access to blood transfusions:

which are critical for managing sickle cell disease. Many rural areas lack blood banks or transportation to larger cities where blood banks are available. This means that people living with sickle cell disease in these areas often go without the transfusions they need, leading to serious complications and even death. Not only that the myths and false beliefs surrounding blood donation and blood transfusion are huge. In 2019, I watched a warrior die because the family rejected blood transfusion and there was nothing we could do. I have also witnessed where some parents refused to donate blood because they believed they didn't have enough blood to give despite the lab test results saying otherwise. This also increases the mortality rate in sickle cell disease.

Traditional Beliefs and Superstitions

In addition to the lack of medical resources, traditional beliefs and superstitions about sickle cell disease were also a major barrier to effective care. Many people in rural communities believed that sickle cell disease was caused by witchcraft or a curse, rather than a genetic disorder. This led to widespread stigmatization and discrimination against people with sickle cell disease, as well as a reluctance to seek medical care. Children with sickle cell disease are still excluded from school or social events, and adults may face difficulty finding work or getting married. This social stigma is also linked to high child mortality rates in rural areas. Many families believe that sickle cell children are a burden on their households and may not seek out medical treatment until it is too late. As a result, children with sickle cell disease in rural areas have a higher risk of death before the age of five compared to those in urban areas.

High Child Mortality Rates

Perhaps the most tragic consequence of the challenges faced by people with sickle cell disease in rural areas was the high child mortality rate. In many villages, children with sickle cell disease die before the age of five, often from preventable complications like infections or malaria. The lack of medical resources, coupled with traditional beliefs and superstitions, meant that many parents did not seek medical care for their sick children until it was too late.

Despite these challenges, there were also signs of hope. In some communities, local organizations and support groups had sprung up to provide assistance and advocacy for people with sickle cell disease. These groups worked tirelessly to raise awareness about sickle cell disease, dispel myths and superstitions, and connect people with medical resources and care.

Late Diagnosis and the Perils of Ignorance:

Sickle cell disease is a genetic condition that affects millions of people worldwide, including many living in rural communities in Nigeria. One of the biggest challenges facing sickle cell patients in these areas is the late diagnosis of the disease, which can lead to a range of health complications and a tragically high child mortality rate.

In many cases, sickle cell disease is not diagnosed until a child starts to exhibit symptoms, which can be months or even years after birth. This is especially true in rural communities, where access to quality healthcare and specialized diagnostic tools may be limited. As a result, many sickle cell patients in these areas do not receive the care and treatment they need until it is too late.

But even when sickle cell disease is diagnosed, there is often a dangerous lack of awareness and education about the condition in rural communities. Many people in these areas do not understand the nature of sickle cell disease and may hold harmful beliefs and myths about the condition. This can lead to a dangerous delay in seeking medical help and can even result in people turning to alternative sources of healing, such as churches or herbalist houses, for assistance.

Overall, the challenges faced by those living with sickle cell disease in rural areas are numerous and complex. Addressing these challenges will require a multifaceted approach that includes increasing access to medical resources, providing education about the disease, dispelling harmful myths and beliefs, and reducing social stigma and discrimination. To address this crisis, we must work to raise awareness about sickle cell disease in rural communities and to provide education and resources to those who need it most. We must work to ensure that sickle cell patients in these areas have access to quality healthcare and specialized diagnostic tools, and that they receive the care and treatment they need as early as possible.

But perhaps most importantly, we must work to combat the ignorance and harmful beliefs that surround sickle cell disease in rural communities. We must work to educate people about the nature of the condition, to dispel harmful myths, and to encourage people to seek medical help when they need it. We must work to create a culture of understanding and acceptance around sickle cell disease so that all people - regardless of where they live - can live a healthy and fulfilling life.

As an organization, the Ignite Sickle Cell Initiative is committed to raising awareness about sickle cell disease in rural communities, and to providing education and resources to those who need it most. We are working to combat ignorance and harmful beliefs and to connect sickle cell patients in rural areas with the care and treatment they need to thrive. But we cannot do this alone. We need the support of individuals, organizations, and governments around the world to come together to address this crisis and to ensure that every child can live a healthy and fulfilling life.

Similarities and Differences
Similarities Between Sickle Cell in Urban and Rural Communities

Despite the significant differences in the challenges faced by people with sickle cell disease in urban and rural communities, there are still some similarities that exist. One of the most significant similarities is the fact that people with sickle cell disease in both urban and rural areas face stigmatization and discrimination. They are often labelled as "sticklers" and ostracized from their communities, which can have a detrimental effect on their mental health and quality of life. This stigma can also lead to discrimination in education and employment opportunities, perpetuating the cycle of poverty that affects many sickle cell patients. Moreover, the lack of awareness and understanding of sickle cell disease in both urban and rural areas contributes to this stigmatization.

Another similarity between sickle cell in urban and rural communities is the high cost of medical care. Many people with sickle cell disease in both areas struggle to afford the necessary medical treatment, which can lead to untreated pain crises and other complications. This can be especially challenging for those in rural communities, who may have limited access to healthcare facilities and have to travel long distances to receive care.

The most notable of these is the emotional toll that sickle cell disease takes on patients and their families Living with sickle cell disease is not only physically painful, but it can also be emotionally draining. The uncertainty of when the next crisis will occur, the financial strain of medical expenses, and the constant worry about the future can take a significant toll on the mental health of patients and their families.

Differences Between Sickle Cell in Urban and Rural Communities

While there are some similarities between sickle cell in urban and rural communities, there are also significant differences. One of the most significant differences is the availability of medical facilities and resources. In urban areas, there are often more medical facilities and resources available, such as specialist clinics and well-equipped hospitals, which can provide better treatment for people with sickle cell disease. In contrast, rural communities often have limited access to healthcare facilities, and those that do exist may lack the necessary resources and trained medical personnel to treat sickle cell disease effectively.

Another difference between sickle cell in urban and rural communities is the influence of traditional beliefs and superstitions. In many rural communities, sickle cell disease is still viewed as a curse or punishment from the gods, and people may turn to traditional healers instead of seeking medical treatment. This can lead to delayed or inadequate care, which can have serious consequences for people with sickle cell disease.

Furthermore, child mortality rates are higher in rural areas, with many children dying from sickle cell disease before the age of five.

This is partly due to the lack of access to medical care, but also due to other factors, such as malnutrition and poor sanitation.

Overall, while there are some similarities between sickle cell in urban and rural communities, the differences in access to medical facilities, resources, and traditional beliefs can have a significant impact on the lives of people with sickle cell disease. It is crucial that these differences are addressed to ensure that everyone with sickle cell disease has access to the necessary care and support to live a full and healthy life

Improving Sickle Cell Care in Nigeria

As I continued to advocate for those living with sickle cell disease, I became acutely aware of the pressing need for improved care and support for patients across Nigeria. The challenges faced by people living with sickle cell in both urban and rural areas were staggering, and it was clear that concerted efforts were needed at all levels to make a positive impact.

The Importance of Policies and Government Involvement

One of the key areas for improvement was in government policies and involvement in the care of sickle cell patients. It was clear that the Nigerian government had a responsibility to prioritize the health and well-being of its citizens, and this was particularly true for those living with chronic illnesses like sickle cell disease.

I am working tirelessly to advocate for increased government funding and support for sickle cell care and research. I met with government officials at local and state levels and there is a plan to take it up to the federal level and make the case for why investment in sickle cell was so critical.

I would love to also work with other patient advocates to draft policy proposals and recommendations for how the government could better support people living with sickle cell in Nigeria.

Implementing Newborn Screening Programs

Another critical area for improvement was in newborn screening programs. As I mentioned, many sickle cell patients are not diagnosed until later in life, which can lead to serious complications and even premature death. However, with the advent of newborn screening tests, it is possible to identify sickle cell disease in infants and begin treatment early, greatly improving outcomes.

So far, we have screened 100 children in rural communities between the ages of 0 to 5 this is to help reduce late diagnosis occurrence and children living with sickle cell were immediately given attention and resources. I hope to work with government officials, Policymakers and other Sickle cell Organizations to help work on getting newborn screening bills.

Increasing Public Awareness and Education

Another critical component of improving sickle cell care in Nigeria was increasing public awareness and education about the disease. Many Nigerians, particularly those in rural areas, do not understand sickle cell and its causes, symptoms, and treatments. This can lead to stigma, discrimination, and even abuse of sickle cell patients.

I worked with schools, community groups, and religious organizations to develop educational programs and materials about sickle cell disease. I also organized public events, such as walks and community medical outreaches which have reached 14 communities to raise awareness about the disease and promote healthy living for those living with sickle cell.

Providing Access to Affordable Medical Care and Resources

Access to affordable medical care and resources was also a major issue for sickle cell patients in Nigeria. Many patients struggle to afford basic medical care, let alone specialized treatments and interventions. This can lead to worsening health outcomes and reduced quality of life.

Presently, We run a monthly clinic that supports over 9 communities to access free routine medications, and resources and educate the caregivers and people living with sickle cell to manage their health better.

I worked with some hospitals, and clinics to secure access to affordable medical care and resources for sickle cell patients. We are working with NHIS and Ondo State Health Insurance Agency to help people living with sickle cell access affordable care at the local level.

Advocacy Efforts and Support Groups

Finally, advocacy efforts and support groups were critical for improving sickle cell care in Nigeria. Patients and their families must feel supported and empowered to speak out about their needs and concerns. They also need access to networks of other patients and families who can offer guidance and support.

I worked with other patient advocates and support groups to develop programs and initiatives to empower sickle cell patients and their families. This included support groups, counselling services, and online resources. We have a lot of support groups on Facebook and WhatsApp in Nigeria presently. Last year, I hosted the first Sickle Cell Caregivers summit to empower caregivers on how to manage their children and the challenges they face. This led to the establishment of the Sickle Cell Caregivers Community. A Facebook group where Caregivers can receive resources and support. Some of our Support Groups include the Sickle Cell Celebs Facebook group, Thriving with Sickle Cell, and the Club is still standing. And we also have a lot more.

It is time to extend this by working with government officials and other stakeholders to advocate for policies and programs that improve care and support for sickle cell patients across Nigeria.

In conclusion, much work still needs to be done to improve sickle cell care in Nigeria. However, I remain hopeful and committed to the cause. There is a critical need for increased support and advocacy for people living with sickle cell disease in Nigeria. This includes improving access to medical care and resources, implementing newborn screening programs, and increasing public awareness and education. It also means challenging traditional beliefs and superstitions that often lead to discrimination and stigma towards those with sickle cell disease.

Through collective efforts and advocacy, I believe we can create a better future for people living with sickle cell disease in Nigeria. I hope this book will serve as a call to action for individuals, communities, and policymakers to prioritize the needs and well-being of those with sickle cell disease.

Making a Difference as an Individual

It is easy to feel helpless in the face of a disease like sickle cell, but you can make a difference as an individual. Every little bit counts and there are several ways in which you can contribute to the fight against sickle cell.

Educate Yourself

The first step in making a difference is to educate yourself about sickle cell. Learn about the disease, its symptoms, and the challenges faced by those living with it. This knowledge will enable you to understand the impact of the disease on individuals and communities and the importance of addressing the issue.

Raise Awareness

Raising awareness about sickle cell is crucial in reducing stigma and improving the lives of those living with the disease. You can start by sharing your story with others, organizing events or campaigns, using social media to spread awareness, or joining a local or international sickle cell organization. Every effort counts and can help to change attitudes and perceptions about sickle cell.

Donate

Donating to sickle cell organizations is a great way to support the fight against the disease. Your donations can help fund research, support programs, and advocacy efforts aimed at improving the lives of those living with sickle cell. Consider donating to local or international organizations like Ignite Sickle Cell Initiative or SAMI, Audrey Sickle Cell Foundation and many more

Volunteer

Volunteering your time and skills is another way to make a difference. You can volunteer at local sickle cell organizations, hospitals, or community events to support awareness campaigns, help patients, or assist with fundraising events. Your time and skills can make a significant impact on the lives of those affected by sickle cell.

Advocate

Advocacy is essential in driving policy change and ensuring that the voices of those affected by sickle cell are heard. As an individual, you can advocate for sickle cell awareness and the needs of those living with the disease by writing letters to policymakers, participating in advocacy campaigns, or engaging with your local government representatives. Your advocacy efforts can help bring about change and improve the lives of sickle cell patients.

In conclusion, every individual has the power to make a difference in the fight against sickle cell. By educating yourself, raising awareness, donating, volunteering, and advocating, you can contribute to the global effort to improve the lives of sickle cell patients.

Reflection On Personal Journey With Sickle Cell

As I come to the end of this, I cannot help but reflect on my personal journey with sickle cell. Reflecting on my journey with sickle cell, I am filled with mixed emotions. On one hand, I feel grateful for the experiences and lessons that have shaped me into who I am today.

On the other hand, I cannot ignore the pain, isolation, and discrimination that I have faced as a result of this condition.

Growing up, I struggled with feelings of inadequacy and self-doubt, wondering why I had to be burdened with a condition that made me different from everyone else. However, as I grew older, I realized that my struggles were not in vain. They have given me a unique perspective and a strong sense of purpose to make a difference in the lives of others living with sickle cell. Through my work with the Ignite Sickle Cell Initiative, I have seen the impact that awareness and education can have on improving the lives of people with sickle cell disease in Nigeria.

Call To Action For Increased Support And Advocacy

To all those reading this book, I urge you to join me in advocating for increased support for people living with sickle cell in Nigeria. We cannot allow ourselves to be complacent in the face of this devastating disease. We must push for better policies, increased funding, and greater awareness. We must work together to ensure that every person living with sickle cell has access to the care and support they need to live a healthy and fulfilling life.

Hope For A Better Future For People Living With Sickle Cell In Nigeria

Despite the challenges we face, I remain hopeful for the future of sickle cell in Nigeria. I have seen firsthand the incredible resilience and strength of people living with this condition, and I know that we can overcome any obstacle that comes our way. With increased advocacy, better policies, and greater awareness, I believe that we can create a brighter future for everyone living with sickle cell in Nigeria. I envision a Nigeria where people living with sickle cell have access to quality healthcare, where they are not discriminated against or stigmatized, and where their contributions to society are valued and celebrated. I believe that this future is possible, but it will take a collective effort from all of us to make it a reality.

As I close this chapter, and indeed this book, I am reminded of the words of Nelson Mandela: "It always seems impossible until it's done." Let us work together to make the impossible possible for people living with sickle cell in Nigeria.

Thank you for taking this journey with me.

A Sickle Cell Journey of Hope and Resilience
By Agness Chitambi

Hello, my name is Agness Chitanda, I would like to tell you how sickle cell has impacted me and my family. I will be telling this story for the first time because, in the past, I was afraid of rejection, isolation, or the stigma I would face if I told people about it. Just to be clear, am not a patient living with sickle cell and am not sure if am a carrier either because I have not shown any symptoms or I have not taken any tests yet. However, my immediate elder sister is a patient living with sickle cell and my little nephew who is only two years old. My sister was declared a sickle cell patient at the early age of five months old while my nephew was declared a patient living with sickle cell at the age of seven months old. The lives of these two individuals have not been easy including family members and their loved ones.

Allow me to explain a little about what sickle cell is and its effects on a patient living with it. Sickle cell can be defined as a blood disorder marked by defective haemoglobin. It can also be defined as an inherited disease in which the red blood cells have an abnormal crescent shape. Sickle cells tend to stick together, blocking small blood vessels, and thereby causing painful and damaging complications. From the definition above, you can tell that sickle cell is an inherited disease which is something you inherited from your parents, it's an inborn disease that you got from your parents when you were born. You can get sickle cell from your friend or partner, like HIV/AIDS or tuberculosis. The following are some of the effects of sickle cell, stroke, blindness, acute chest pains, leg ulcers, organ damage, pulmonary hypertension, gallstones and many others. The signs or symptoms of sickle cell start showing in the patient at the early age of five months or six, it varies from one patient to another.

My sister started showing signs or symptoms at five months old. Being in a village set-up, it took very long for my parents to know what it was, so instead of taking her to the hospital for a check-up, they took her to traditional healers and gave her traditional herbs, believing she was bewitched. In my village, people used to believe so much in witchcraft than natural illness, in fact, to them, when one gets seriously ill suddenly, they believed that someone bewitched that person. After my sister was not responding or getting healed from the traditional herbs, my parents finally decided to take her to the hospital. After doing several tests, the doctors told my parents that my sister was diagnosed with sickle cell and this news didn't sit well with my parents. To them, as far as they were concerned, she was bewitched by someone in the village. They were in denial to the extent that they had to talk to a lot of councillors to make them understand what was going on. It took a while for them to understand the fact their little daughter had sickle cell, a long-life disease and she had to be on medication for the rest of her life. This was the worst news I had ever encountered, the hospital was very far from home, and my parents were small-scale farmers who never even had enough food to feed the family, as if the suffering they were going through was not enough, they now had a child living with sickle cell who needed special medical care and hospital was very far from home. It was the worst nightmare and the only thing my mom could do was to cry and hope for a miracle from the Lord.

To be kept alive, my sister had to be medicated, but even with the medication present and being taken according to the doctor's prescription, she would still get seriously sick suddenly and end up admitted to a hospital. This used to happen on several occasions, especially when she was young, my poor parents who were small-scale farmers who never even had enough food, had no choice but to work in people's maize or cotton fields to earn money for my sister's medication and transport to and from the hospital. Because of being medicated and admitted most of the time, she grew at a very slower pace and most people in the village made fun of her. When she was enrolled in school, the situation which ugly already became worse, this was because our school was located nearly three kilometres from home, and walking this distance did not sit well with her health issues. Her legs would get swollen, sometimes she used to faint out of nowhere being the only sibling that she had at that time, I had no choice but to carry her whenever she said that she was tired. She used to have episodes of sharp pains, which would leave her hospitalised or at home for days, sometimes weeks and she missed school during this whole period. I remember this one time when were in grade six, she was admitted to the hospital for the whole month, and she missed school this whole time. My sister was a slow learner already, missing school for a long time because she was admitted to a hospital or sick at home made her school performance even worse. She wasn't doing well at school; hence, she kept repeating grades and this whole situation led to her being bullied by pupils and some teachers who never knew her sickness. She became antisocial, depressed, and suicidal. She blamed herself for failing and thought that it was her fault that she was sick. She used to tell me that she would be happy if she just passed away and this made me very sad. I would pray that she would be healed and cry myself to sleep. I didn't like seeing my sister sick, being bullied, or isolated, all of these made me feel sad. So as long she was around, I would sit next to her just to let her know that she's not alone and that I love her more than anything in the world. When her performance in school was not improving, my mom went to school and begged teachers to help her with extra lessons and some notes whenever she missed school. This move did the trick, it helped her to improve a little bit. My mother also told some teachers about my sister's sickle cell problem, most of them became nice to her and encouraged her by making her realize that she wasn't the only sickle cell patient and that with hard work and determination, she can be anything she wanted to be. I was very happy for the first time seeing my sister being strong and determined. Even though she was mostly in and out of hospitals, this time around she started socializing a little bit and made a few friends. I was so happy for her and so was my mom and my entire family members. Her life took a positive turn and she decided to fight for a happy life despite her illness.

A few years later, she completed school and decided to study nursing, I was the happiest, the whole family supported her decision, and she went to college. While at college, she met a man who fell in love with her and without wasting time, she got pregnant and dropped out of college. Unfortunately, she made a huge mistake of not telling the man about her sickle cell diagnosis during dating. In the first weeks of pregnancy, she kept hiding that she was sick, and the husband noticed that she would, faint frequently and get episodes of shape pains. So, he decided to take her to the hospital for check-ups and he was old, she had a high-risk pregnancy because she was a sickle cell patient. He was very disappointed to the extent that he brought her back to my mom's house. We as a family were not happy that she decided to hide such kind of sensitive information from her partner, but we felt sorry seeing her in that state, begging her husband not to leave her. It was very sad, and I felt sad seeing my mom comforting her precious daughter who was crying uncontrollably, it was very sad. We were once again taken back to old sad days when happiness was nowhere to be seen. How I wished she was a little more honest to avoid this tragedy, but it was too late. According to her, she had to lie because she was afraid that he would leave her, in fact, her insecurities made her do it. All I could do at this time to listen to her and tell her that she was special to me and our entire family. Days passed and her husband came back even though his family didn't support him. Being a high-risk pregnancy, she needed some expensive medicine prescribed by the doctors. Her husband wasn't working, so my mom had to pay for her medical bills, it was hard. I had to look for a job to help but even with all of these efforts, she ended up losing the baby in the seventh month. It was a sad experience for all of us but to her am sure it was worse. My mother was much stressed, she cried a lot because she could not stand seeing her daughter going through all of this after everything she did. It was really depressing I remember questioning myself over and over why my family had to go through all of this, but it was a senseless question because no one answered me. However, the doctors assured my sister that she's able to have children as long as she starts attending antenatal in the early stages if her pregnancy. This was good news to us, especially her because she always wanted to have a baby. After a year, she got pregnant and lost the baby despite doing everything the doctor recommended, she became desperate to have a child, so she got pregnant again and she lost the baby again. This time, the doctor advised that she should not be pregnant because it was very risky, and she might lose her life if she tried to have a child again.

It was very hard for all of us to accept this news, my sister who was already in pain and depressed could not process this news properly. The thought of her husband leaving her because she could not have children drove her crazy. She became suicidal once again. She attempted to take her life on several occasions. I dropped everything I was doing to be close to her and make sure she was not trying to hurt herself. Her husband became very distant because, at this point, most of his family members advised him just to leave her because she was not able to give him any kids. He almost took their advice but later, he changed his mind. During this whole time of misfortune, my sister used to tell me how much she loved her husband and how she never wanted to lose him. It was heartbreaking but I had to stay strong and assure her that he wouldn't leave her even though I had no idea that he would ever come back for her. At this moment, I hated sickle cell disease more than ever and I was so frustrated and depressed. I wished for a lot of things, but none came true. Once again, we were back to square and I could not do anything to help my sister or my poor mum who was in so much sorrow at this point, the only thing I did was to watch them cry hopelessly. Deep down, I didn't have the strength to comfort her, but I had to play the strong super sister and whenever she wasn't around, I would cry bitterly. I really did hope for a miracle a million times during these hopeless moments, but it was all in vain. My family and I had to pull ourselves together so we could encourage my sister to get back on her feet. Her husband luckily came back into her life, and we helped each other to encourage her, and she started improving, with time she was once again back on her feet. It was so exciting to see this. It brought a lot of happiness to my family. Because sickle cell is a lifelong disease and is incurable, my sister till now is still diagnosed with it but the good news is that she no longer faints frequently like she used to when she was pregnant. She still gets the episodes of pain sometimes, but they are not frequent either. She's much better now.

I wish this could have been the end of sickle cell's impacts on my family but no, this disease wasn't done with us yet, two years ago, they welcomed their first baby, a bouncing baby boy. They were so happy and so was the rest of the entire family. I mean who would not be happy after so much misfortune that we went through. Unfortunately, our happiness lasted only for less than six months when the baby became seriously ill and started showing signs or symptoms of sickle cell. We didn't want to believe it, but we had no choice, when the baby was taken to the hospital the doctors confirmed it was sickle cell after doing their examinations. This time around things were a little different because the boy was taken to the hospital earlier unlike in my sister's case. The treatment started on time and there were less complications. I was happy and grateful for the way my brother handled the situation because, unlike my parents, he didn't believe in witchcraft that much. During the second case of sickle cell, my family and I had learnt a lot about this disease so there wasn't so much panic, and our finances were not that bad, so we helped my brother whenever he needed our help. It was another terrible tragedy that my family had to experience again.

I would not say that *everything was easy this time around* but again it was not as hard as the first time either. Because during the first case, we had no knowledge about the disease and that made it more difficult to deal with. We even had a rural clinic in our village, so instead of travelling long distances to the hospital to get medical care, we would only go to the clinic unless the situation was bad. It is a sad experience to have a patient living with sickle cell because they might be okay in one minute and critically ill the next minute or even faint just out of nowhere. Until now, I don't understand how this happens, but I wish sickle cell could be cured completely because seeing my little nephew admitted to the clinic from time to time was so traumatizing, it is an experience that I would not wish on my worst enemy. I will never get used to it; the pain is unbearable. It has brought a lot of harm to me and my family.

Sickle cell indeed brought a lot of harm in my family, here are some of the negative impacts it imposed on us, during the time my sister was declared a sickle cell patient, my parents had no knowledge about sickle cell, they became so depressed, they had no money nor enough food to feed the family, in fact, there was poverty. They were going through a lot just to put food on the table, receiving the news of their first baby girl being diagnosed with a disease that was not curable was the worst news they could ever get. It brought them to their knees. Our home was stricken by poverty, they had to work in other people's fields just to find food to eat, and sometimes we would sleep without eating anything at all. Most of the time, they missed my sister's medical appointments because they didn't have transport money to go to the hospital. The level of poverty became worse because now they had to find money for my sister's medication and transport to and from the hospital. It was a difficult time for all of us. I remember going to school barefoot because there was no money to buy shoes. It was very cold and most children who were my age had shoes even stockings, they laughed at me, while some even mocked and bullied me. That did not bother me a lot because I knew my parents had a lot of problems and did not have money, so I continued going to school. My entire family was subjected to mockery and bullying due to the fact that most people in my village had no knowledge about sickle cell disease, they discriminated against us because according to them, we were cursed, or my parents were witches who wanted to kill their own daughter. Many people thought that this disease was contagious, so they stopped coming to our house and stopped their children from playing with us, we were isolated almost completely, it was so depressing. We were badly discriminated against to the extent that we felt like outcasts in our very own village. It was the worst experience that I don't want to go through ever again. The impacts of bullying and mockery left my sister with little trust in humanity. She's afraid to open up because she's scared of being judged. We never had a chance to save money or improve our lives because it was always a problem after another problem. We had to survive each day.

By the grace of the Lord, we survived this ugly experience and today, I feel like it was indeed an ugly a terrible experience, but we had to go through it to have a better a better understanding and knowledge about sickle cell. Today, can stand up against all kinds of discrimination against sickle cell patients which I doubt I could have been able to do if I never had the first-hand experience. When my sister was going through a hard d time of losing babies from one to another, when she was on the verge of losing her marriage because of sickle cell disease which made her have complicated pregnancies and give birth to stillborn babies, our hopes and dreams were shuttered.

I tried to help whenever I could but seeing my sister crying always, made me become so depressed and there was nothing I could do to help her. Sometimes, I used to think that we would never be happy in our lives. I almost dropped out of school at some point because all of my friends had nice shoes and school uniforms. The bullying was just too much sometimes, I never had many friends because I was the dirty kid without shoes or a proper uniform. They never bothered to ask me about my home situation, they just laughed at me. It was so painful. All I wanted was someone to talk to me or just ask me what was wrong, but no one cared. They laughed but they didn't care to ask why I was this miserable and dirty little child. Seeing my sick sister being bullied, mocked, and laughed at added to my sorrow, I became a sadist at a young age. I wished more people could understand that my sister was just a victim of a genetic disease that she had no control over. I had no one to share my sad stories with so I cried myself to sleep almost every night.

Today, I wish to see a lot of activists talking about sickle cell a lot in my village. Most people especially villagers have no idea of what sickle cell is, so when someone is affected, they react negatively which is not okay for the patient, or all the people related to the patient. I want more villagers to be empowered with knowledge about different diseases and teach them about the effects of discrimination and isolation of patients. They do it because of ignorance and their traditional beliefs. I have seen a lot of HIV/AIDS activists in my village but sickle cell? I have not seen one not even a single day. People need to learn what sickle cell is so that discrimination and stigma can be avoided at all costs. I don't want to see another family going through what I went through, it's not okay. It hurts seeing a patient being discriminated against, isolated, or mocked when they are supposed to be loved and cared for by people who are not sick. My sister would have lost her life because my parents didn't know what sickle cell is and it took long for them to take her to hospital which was very risky considering her state of health then. At first, they did not accept that their daughter was diagnosed with sickle cell because they had no knowledge about the disease but when they were taught what it was, they agreed to treatment which shows that knowledge is needed for people to make the right decisions. I strongly believe that if we talk more and educate more people about sickle cell, all this discrimination can go away in no time. Let us work together and change the narrative. This has been my story about sickle cell and how it has impacted me and my family. Thanks for reading.

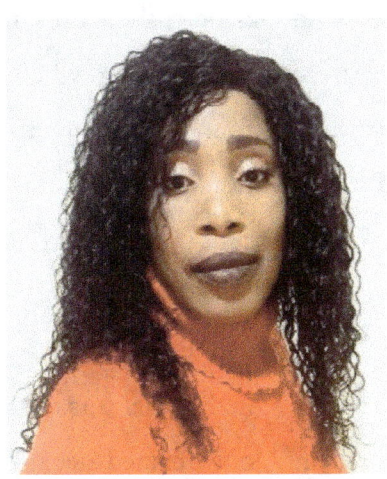

Fighting the Silent Battle: A Story of a Warrior
By Lillian Chikuta

Born in 1980 17th of January at Kitwe Central Hospital. Am a sickle cell patient and warrior. I was born in a family of 5, 4 girls and 1 boy. Our firstborn has no sickle cell, the second born of our family who happens to be me has sickle cell, our third born has no sickle cell, our fourth born equally had cell and she's late now because of it and finally, our last born is sickle cell free.

After falling very ill at 3 months old and upon discovering I had swollen fingers on my hand, I was immediately rushed to Kitwe Central Hospital by my parents, after being examined by doctors they could not determine what exactly was wrong with me.

My parents instead opted for alternative solutions to my predicament, they sought out for herbalist but nothing changed and I was finally spotted unwell by a certain lady on the bus we were on with my parents, who suggested I should be rushed back to Kitwe Central Hospital and gave my parents a specific ward where I was supposed to be taken, upon arrival, we found a certain male Doctor from Uganda, and a second round of tests were done this time around the results were different, the doctor discovered I had sickle cell anaemia, and I was instantly placed on medication.

At the age of 5, my blood level was very low and the doctors suggested I do a blood transfusion, but that was not meant to happen as during the procedure, my blood reacted negatively with foreign blood and it started coming out of my nose and ears and doctors deduced that a blood transfusion was not feasible at that particular time, as my system couldn't accept foreign blood and later suggested, that I should just drink and eat foods rich in zinc in order to boost my blood levels.

At the age of 12, I suffered from yellow fever, my eyes were yellowish in colour, and I became extremely weak, my parents and I visited the hospital and unfortunately, we were not given any medication for yellow fever, the healthcare providers had advised that I take water mixed with sugar and on certain intervals, I ate sugarcane as advised. After a combination of these food stuffs, I finally overcame yellow fever, since the incident, I stayed for a period of 9 years without having any complications or sickle cell crisis or pain in my body. At the age of 17, I found a job as a babysitter for a period, a job I carried out passionately for a period of 8 years. However, the journey was not without its own challenges, during the period I worked as a babysitter, I seriously got ill at the age of 21, to the point of being admitted to the University teaching hospital, for two weeks, upon being discharged from hospital, few moments after I arrived back home, I fainted again and I was subsequently returned to the hospital for further treatment and I stayed for 3 days more at the hospital before I was discharged for a second time. After that, I stayed for 7 years straight without having pain or crisis in my body.

Then I found another job in the industries under a certain company that was into selling artificial hair, I worked with them for a year until my blood level dropped due to the hot environments we were working under.

This time around, I really needed the blood transfusion if I was to survive the brutal phase of my life, however, not every doctor understood my predicament as a certain named Doctor at the University teaching hospital said I was faking my illness and he said I should be sent back home. This statement had left me and my family entirely disappointed and both my parents were extremely depressed by the Doctor's utterances towards my illness, my mother had thought I would die as a result of being sent back home in my worst state, and the entire family expressed their deepest disappointment because none of them had expected such words of mockery to come from a healthcare provider, that was on a Friday afternoon and I was returned to the hospital on Monday morning the following week. After being accessed by a different doctor, eventually, I was admitted to the hospital.

Unlike the previous attempt to carry out a blood transfusion which failed, this time around, at the age of 28, I had a successful blood transfusion after that I was given morphine and later discharged even though I told the doctors that I was unwell but that plea was not heeded to, I was discharged anyway and while at home, the effects of morphine kicked in and I was extremely weak for a period of 8 months and I could barely do anything by my own, but I continued to visit the hospital for a regular check-up and the doctors confirmed that morphine badly reacted with my system hence weakness, but the medication was not anything out of the ordinary, I was given folic acid and Delta prime.

Until I got better, then I started working for a certain Chinese clothing company, in town, three years later at the same company, I suffered from chest acute syndrome and I was admitted for a period of 1 month and two weeks, I was later discharged and after a month of recovering from home, I later resumed with work at the same Chinese clothing company and after a week of working uninterrupted, on a particular day after having a great work day, I was going back home before I got hit by a fast-moving vehicle on my left leg, Subsequently, I developed endless pain for on my left leg, the pain came directly from my hip area,

After months of visiting the clinic at the University teaching hospital, concerning the same sharp pain I had, I was advised to start using crutches, because doctors couldn't exactly determine what was causing the pain. I had continued reporting for work with my crutches, after a period of 5 years, doctors finally discovered I had developed avascular necrosis of the hip.

The only possible solution to that according to orthopaedic surgeons is hip replacement surgery, and in 2015, I was supposed to undergo a hip replacement surgery but unfortunately, I couldn't afford the quoted price and as a result, having a hip replacement was not possible. After working with the Chinese clothing company for a period of 10 years, I finally stopped working with them in 2018 due to the pain of travelling to and from work with crutches.

In 2019, I got very sick, and I was in deep pain because of the same, I had to endure sleepless nights till this day, and my leg gives me a lot of pain from time to time,

In 2022, I got seriously sick of yellow fever, and I was admitted to the hospital for a period of one week, until I was given my second blood transfusion, since then several tests have confirmed that both my liver and kidneys have developed certain complications, however, the complications are not that severe.

From 2022 to the present, I have taken hydroxyurea, B12 vitamins and vitamin C.

Looking at how I had frequently experienced sickle cell crisis and other body pains, Doctors had decided to place me on hydroxyurea, which is very expensive on my part because I don't often buy the medication because of its price tag, but whenever I buy and take it, I rarely experience sickle cell crisis and I gain a lot of weight because of the medication, I don't have any side effects, it works perfectly for me.

Sickle cell has really affected my love life, whenever I find myself in a relationship and I disclose to them my condition, they gradually withdraw away from me and end up breaking up the relationship and according to others, they think a person with sickle cell can't bear healthy children. It is because of this societal falsehood that has made a lot of men see me as person living with sickle cell unworthy to them. And up to now, I have no children neither am I married, however, I do find my consolation from God and family, most of them understand my condition and render their support whenever and however they can, other family members, however, still think my illness has never been real and I have been faking it all along, others say I'm just a lazy person.

Sickle cell has really drained my family financially, as it strikes impromptu and they have to find money immediately, so I'm quickly rushed to the hospital for medical attention and buy certain prescribed medication from private pharmacies.

Despite all the pain and hurdles, I have endured, I have a total of 43 years and counting.

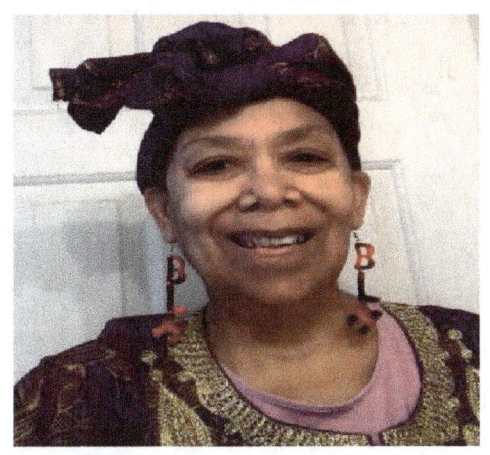

Aging Sickle Cell Patients.
By Linda Armstead

When I was diagnosed with Sickle Cell Anaemia, the doctors told my mother my life expectancy was 16 years of age. I am very fortunate and happy to say I am 64 years old and will turn 65 in September of this year, 2023. The number of older patients with Sickle Cell is steadily increasing. Though still not a large number it seems as though many Sickle Cell Doctors have limited information on various treatment plans for their senior patients.

I will use myself as an example. There are many Paediatric Sickle Cell Doctors but when you transition to adult doctors, the choices are far fewer. I stayed with the doctor I had when I was 15 because he provided care for both paediatric and adult patients. When he retired, I was in my 20s I asked him to refer me to an adult doctor. He couldn't recommend anyone, so I went to another hospital. The adult doctor at the new hospital only had a few Sickle Cell patients. He mainly saw oncology patients and after a few years of seeing me, he totally gave up all his sickle cell patients and only saw Oncology patients. I began a research study with the doctors at NIH and didn't have a Haematology doctor I routinely saw the Haematologist at NIH. They put me on Hydroxyurea as part of the study or clinical trial. Hydroxyurea is a cancer drug that is used with Sickle Cell patients by helping to prevent the formation of sickle-shaped red blood cells. It reduces pain episodes and the need for blood transfusions.

A large number of Sickle Cell patients take Hydroxyurea with much success. My niece who also has Sickle Cell takes it and leads a productive life. Some sickle cell patients like me, suffer from the side effects of the drug. At the time I was working, and I told the doctors I had to stop the study because the side effects were affecting me adversely, it interfered with my ability to work. I left NIH and if I had a pain crisis, I would go to the ER.

As a Sickle Cell patient, I have had horrible experiences going to the ER, so I no longer go. One example of my bad experience is when I was about 35 and went to the ER, the doctors were changing shifts and though they pulled the curtain, they were discussing my case right on the other side of that curtain. Dr. A (the leaving Dr.) Stated - "She claims she is having a Sickle Cell crisis, but she doesn't act like the other sickle cell patients. I think she just wants attention so do a psychiatric work-up on her." Dr. B (the next shift doctor), "OK, so I will call the psychiatrist on call tonight." When Dr. B, pulled the curtain back to enter my area, I proceeded to lay him out, letting him know I could hear the conversation and the other doctor had no right to accuse me of lying and all he had to do was perform a CBC and he would see my Haemoglobin and Haematocrit would be low. Dr. B apologized and started to treat me with the respect I deserved. I did need and got a transfusion, that was not the last time I went to the ER but after 3 or 4 more times of bad treatments, I no longer go to the ER for any treatments.

I found a new Haematologist who specializes in Sickle Cell Anaemia. She encouraged me to try Hydroxyurea again. Even though it was successful in increasing my Haemoglobin, I was still feeling the side effects that were affecting my ability to work, so once again I stopped taking it. I was put on transfusion therapy after having an aplastic crisis. An aplastic crisis is when your body stops making enough red blood cells to keep up with your body destroying red blood cells. My Haematocrit, which is usually around 23 % dropped to 11%. After getting transfusions to get my levels up, I was put on regular transfusions of 4 times a year.

A few years later, I took a job in NJ and looked for a Haematologist there. I found a Haematologist whose concentration was Sickle Cell. I told the doctor I researched him, and I feel he was offended because I was looking up his credentials when I first saw him. I gave him my history, so he could know about me. He insisted I take Hydroxyurea, and he got mad with me for not wanting to take it after I had tried it twice before and it did not work for me. He said he couldn't see any patient who didn't want to take his advice. So even though he was listed as my doctor, I never saw him again as a patient. He would only have his Residents care for me.

When my job ended in NJ, I moved back to Maryland and went back to the Haematologist I had been before. I started doing travel medical computer training for my work, so getting a transfusion 4 times a year and seeing the doctor 2 times a year worked well for me.

After a few years, the facility opened a Sickle Cell Infusion Centre where I can go if I need a transfusion or fluid infusion. Life on the road is difficult for people with Sickle Cell Anaemia. I am now on disability and have increased the number of blood transfusions I need from 4 times to 6 times a year. My body could not handle the draw of a unit of blood before I started my transfusion. So, now, I have monthly transfusions of one unit of blood a month instead of the 6 times a year with two units of blood. My list of current issues is as follows:

- I now have transfusion-related Iron Overload due to the number of transfusions I get a year.
- I have Stage 2 renal disease that the doctors are trying to help keep from getting worse. (The doctor put me on Lisinopril for the kidneys, not for high blood pressure. But the medicine made me very dizzy so I stopped taking it. I did inform the doctor. Who agreed because I have low to normal blood pressure, the Lisinopril was not helpful.)
- My potassium is high which causes protein in my urine. Indicating kidney damage. I am on a low to no-potassium diet. Which seems to be helping.

- I have Osteoporosis with high calcium and low Vitamin D. But because the calcium in high amounts can also affect the kidneys, I was taken off calcium and any vitamin mixture that includes calcium).
- I had a nodule on my left parathyroid gland that was surgically removed. The surgeon actually had to remove three of the four parathyroid glands because they were all affected, and my calcium and vitamin D levels were returning to normal.
- I have been diagnosed with MGUS - Monoclonal Gammopathy of Undetermined Significance - a condition where an abnormal protein or Monoclonal protein is in your blood. This protein is formed in the bone marrow, and it can cause kidney problems.
- I am being treated for a possible auto-immune disease. (The doctor put me on Hydroxychloroquine. This medicine is to help prevent any worsening and development of auto-immune disease). Even though I am on the lowest dose, it still causes dizziness. As a suggestion from my doctor, I take the medication at night, so I do feel the dizzy effects during the day.

The iron overload in me now has liver involvement and is also in my heart.

The first medication my doctor prescribed for Chelation therapy was too hard on my kidneys and was rejected by my Nephrologist. The second med had a $250 copay per 30-day supply of medicine. The cost of the co-pay was something I could not afford. I found out the company offered financial assistance, so I called them and was told it was only for people who had

Thalassemia with Transfusion Related Iron Overload. When I asked what about people with Sickle Cell Anaemia who have the same issue of transfusion-related Iron Overload, I was told it was because not enough people with Sickle Cell get this so it was excluded from the FDA mandate of who could get financial assistance. The Haematologist informed me it was because they could not get enough Sickle Cell patients in the Clinical Trials. Since many clinical trials are offered that Sickle Cell patients are not aware of, we need to make sure we talk to our doctors about them.

Since the chelation medicine was out of the picture, my doctor suggested Oxbryta by GBT (Global Blood Therapeutics) a medication still in clinical trials, I was told Oxbryta is not a chelation med, but it increases the haemoglobin in a patient which could lead to fewer needs for transfusions. The cost of the co-pay is $200 for a 30-day supply. I still cannot afford this med either. But was told the manufacturer did offer financial assistance. I was lucky, they approved me to get the medication for free with my insurance. My haemoglobin has increased from 7.5 gm/dL to 8.3 gm/dL which is still outside of the normal range for an adult woman of 12 - 17 gm/dL but is a great improvement for me after only 3 weeks of use. The downfall is the side effects I have which were severe diarrhoea and headaches.

Since I could no longer take the Oxbryta, I did qualify for chelation therapy using an infusion pump. The pump was surgically implanted in my chest on the left side. The pump seemed too big when it was placed. I have had it for a year and still have issues with it but my iron level has gone from a high of 2,215 to 822 ng/mL. This is still high with the normal range of 13-150 ng/mL, but it is moving in the right direction. Unfortunately, the pump has caused two blood clots in my heart and I am now on Eliquis, a blood thinner. I asked my doctor how long I would have to be on it and was told as long as I had the pump.

Even though I have sickle cell and issues from it, I still work with The Armstead-Barnhill Foundation, an organization started by my sister one year after her daughter was born with sickle cell, it is an organization that seeks funds to help researchers find a cure for sickle cell. I am also involved with SiNERGe and ECHO, organizations working to bring awareness of sickle cell to the world, and also support patients, organizations, and facilities to bring about improvements in the health of the sickle cell patient.

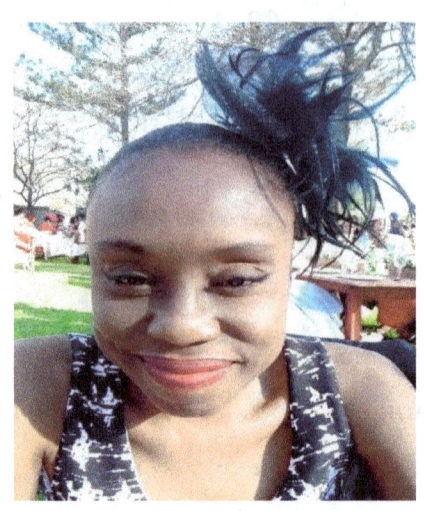

Sickle Cell and Me: Challenges Battle With Silent Disease
By Lusubilo Gondwe

My name is Lusubilo Gondwe. I am a female Broadcast Journalist working with a privately-owned Radio Station called Phoenix FM based in Zambia and specifically in the capital city of Lusaka. I am also a trained Early Educator. I live with a condition called Sickle cell anaemia or SCD an acronym for Sickle cell disease.

My sickle cell diagnosis was made when I was just six months old. My mother tells me, she thought I had malaria initially because one morning, she noticed I had overslept and had to wake me up to feed me, after I threw up the entire meal and my body temperature increased, my parents rushed me to hospital. The doctor after ordering a full blood count and malaria test, discovered I had haemoglobin count of two. I was quickly transfused and later upon further investigation, I was discovered to have sickle cell anaemia. That was the very first of my blood transfusions.

My health was very fine from then on until I reached the age of 31. One Friday, I developed a severe backache and chest pain and had to be hospitalized, the doctor ordered numerous tests and it was discovered that my HB or haemoglobin count was at four, for some reason my body had adapted to low HB and had started compensating by working harder to pump blood around my body.

I was given two pints of blood but had to receive another two when just seven days later my HB had dropped to four again. The tests ordered after my transfusion revealed that 1 had developed a complication of heart failure and tricuspid regurgitation (one of my heart valves had stopped working as well as it should) this meant my HB had to be maintained at steady levels and I was also placed on new drug enalapril for life. Enalapril assists my heart in not working too hard, however, the challenge is maintaining my HB at steady levels, with steady being at least seven. Thankfully, I no longer need to take it and haven't in over five years plus.

I also spent about six years in and out of hospital after every third month or so to receive blood at some point in my life. The highest number of blood pints I have received at a go was about seven years ago when I had a haemolytic crisis (this is when the spleen destroys red blood cells too rapidly and drops the HB very quickly). I was given four pints of blood at a go. My struggles with the frequent need for blood have caused me to have a deep appreciation for blood transfusions and blood donors it was an emotionally taxing period for me and my family. However, their support and the support of blood bank staff and haematologists have helped me endure countless procedures and hospital stays, needing blood so frequently to survive makes one appreciate how vital blood transfusions are as they had literally been my lifeline for a while. I have experienced how blood transfusions restore energy and instantly bring about a feeling of wellness.

I have a lot of gratitude for people running social media groups that discuss sickle cell disease because they provide a vital source of information and knowledge sharing as well as encouragement on coping with complications that arise from living with sickle cell anemia, this is because Zambian adults living with sickle cell anemia have very little knowledge and access to information about complications that may arise as a result of their condition and how to deal with them. It is also a challenge to find blood in blood banks for varied reasons (this can be because of myths surrounding the donating of blood such as the belief that the blood can be used for nefarious reasons such as to bewitch the donor or the idea that those not ready to know their status especially with regards to give may be told what they are not ready to hear, or the church one congregates with forbids blood donations for religious reasons. This has in Zambian set up led to more Students and school-going children being used as the pool from where blood donations are sourced when schools close and children are on recess it means the blood bank will have significant shortages of blood available for transfusions.) So, it is from these online platforms that I have learnt about proper nutrition and some natural ways of avoiding the need for too many medications and boosting my haemoglobin levels naturally. I have for example learnt about molasses, blackstrap molasses and how it helps fight off fatigue and gives energy, if you live with SCD or care for a child or someone living with SCD, you know that fatigue is sometimes a serious battle but since I started using it, I rarely experience fatigue. Molasses also aids with boosting iron when my iron levels are low (contrary to the teaching that people with SCD don't need iron they sometimes do run low on iron).

I have also learnt about juicing or blending fruits and vegetables together and how this helps boost haemoglobin (HB) levels and just generally meets the nutrition needs of the body and one's general wellness.

The necessity for blood transfusions remains crucial, but so is the need for knowledge sharing with the larger community to dispel falsehoods. and it's important to have more blood donors come on board and donate blood, there is in fact a great need in this area (the wider community needs sensitization on how vital blood donations are not just for people living with SCD but even for themselves as medical emergencies are a reality for all because, in times of emergency, blood transfusions can make all the difference between life and death. People need a mindset change and dispel the various myths they have about blood donations; much advocacy is needed in this area and the blood bank requires the assistance of many stakeholders to achieve success in this exercise)

Zambian adults living with SCD face a myriad of challenges from having to eke out a living to being married or caring for a family and the challenges associated with parenting and the pressures of everyday life and living all whilst dealing with their health. It can be a tough balancing act for those who do not live with the condition but is even more burdensome for those who do. Stress is a very real reality of life and a trigger for a crisis in someone with SCD.

The problem with sickle cell disease is that it is not just about pain crisis alone no, it can and does present a host of varied complications as well - so one never knows what complications may come their way but this is why is it important to have access to as much knowledge about the disease as possible and also learn to keep a very healthy lifestyle and diet.

It is just critical for someone with SCD to especially know how to cope with stress whether from the pressures of relating with others and the everyday pressures of life or one's emotions and the stress from everyday tasks.

Presently, Zambia has many who advocate for better treatment in hospitals and health care facilities, for easier access to treatment options like blood transfusions, blood exchange programs, more effective pain management options and better treatment from health care practitioners. These advocates do their best and are doing a good job. However, there is a need too for advocates (and this is not restricted to Zambia but is a challenge for All African nations) to get cheaper access to Bone Marrow Transplants (BMT), Better nutrition, sensitization of the general Zambian populace on the importance of blood donations and dispelling of myths surrounding blood donations, stress management and mindset change and in the area of total wellness, by this, I mean dealing with and overcoming depression which is something many with SCD struggle with as it can be quite debilitating and can really play up with one's health and abilities literally (one can be fine one minute and dealing with a backache, stomach ache or migraine or swelling of fingers or toes the next minute. Periods can be quite a difficult time for many as this is when the crisis will kick in, sudden weather changes, extremes of temperatures or the onset of complications, these can change one day drastically, and one can be grounded when they may be in the middle of needing to get tasks done. It can really pull a number on a person's mental state and cause them to fall into depression because crises can last anywhere from a few minutes or hours to days or even weeks).

This intervention is needed from childhood since many children begin to feel limited in their abilities because they are different from their peers or are unable to perform what their peers do, especially when even care givers, teachers and parents also reinforce the message that a child can't do much. Or the very often recited phrase ' will not live long enough ' to achieve or do anything worthwhile. The pain crisis and frequent hospitalizations also contribute to the thinking that SCD means that one's life is going to be short and gloomy and yet this is simply not true. The problem is, it creates a tendency toward depression in many living with SCD and this is what many struggle with even as adults. It is an unspoken truth. A truth that needs to be tackled and dispelled and with the right tools and education, I believe that this narrative and experience can be overturned for many.

Total wellness also includes but is not limited to, having a positive vision for oneself and life, as well as having an unwavering determination and belief in one's own abilities to get things done and achieve whatever one sets out to do. It also includes knowledge on the use of herbs in achieving wellness, for example, I use cayenne pepper or just red chillies in my food daily and I have stopped having the problem of poor blood circulation, especially in my legs. I used to have a lot of pain in my legs previously. I also discovered that cayenne pepper or just the simple red chillies it is made from also helps in preventing strokes. I have also learned that taking a clove of garlic a day also eliminates blood clots from forming in one's system and am still on my journey or discovery as I seek to have more knowledge of how natural herbs and plants can assist me in keeping well.

This type of knowledge I believe can assist many in learning how to keep healthy naturally and reduce medicine usage.

In my Experience. Life is tough whether one lives with a medical condition or not and this realization made many years ago helped me learn that one's mental attitude is very critical to gaining success or failure in whatever one faces.

Life will throw a lot at us and dealing with sickle cell makes life a lot tougher because you have to consider your health before you can consider anything else. However, everyone must have a coping mechanism and mine has been to develop a tougher mental attitude.

I don't see myself as different from anyone else, I only find different ways of achieving what I need to get done.

It's also been a great game changer for me to discover that with God all things are possible. My trust in God and His ability to get me through and out of anything is ironclad. I know that to be alive is in itself a struggle for all and no one has it easy on this earth but with God, there is so much we can get done and get through.

People living with sickle cell are just regular people but with a greater appreciation for life (hospital stays have a way of changing how one views life completely). In all one endeavours to do; success is guaranteed when God is first sought and fully relied upon. (I haven't had a hospital stay in over five years now and I don't take that lightly and I am just grateful for every day God keeps me fine and away from the need for hospital stays as well as for good health and life).

The power of prayer should not be underestimated especially for those living with SCD and added to that the need to take good care of oneself.

Every person living with SCD should know how to create a balance in their life between playtime, rest and work. They should have a strong belief system and a strong sense of self which parents, care givers and themselves as individuals should build and constantly reinforce.

Every person living with SCD should know their limits and by this, I mean what they can handle workwise and even physically so as not to strain oneself unduly which can cause crisis. They should know their limits in terms of having a personal schedule that regulates their sleep times, how much alcohol they should take if they do take some and how much time to spend on extraneous activities like exercise.

Every person living with sickle cell disease should learn to monitor their bodies, know when they need to relax, know when a crisis is coming on and avoid it if possible before it becomes fully set, know when to get help and always have their medication stock refilled at the right times.

Every person living with sickle cell should understand the importance of embracing a healthy lifestyle and healthy eating habits and learn how to keep well hydrated.

Good hydration is very important in maintaining good health and keeping crises away. I once went into a shock a few years ago because although I was drinking sufficient amounts of water, sufficient being two and half litres of water daily (in my thinking, this was a sufficient amount of water, so I was fine) I was low on electrolytes and also had low Hb.

I was placed on saline solution drips and stayed in the hospital for about four days till I was stabilized, the pain that came with receiving the electrolytes was terrible because I went into a very bad crisis and only pain medications like morphine helped me get relief.

The doctor that attended to me later explained that I would need to be incorporating electrolytes into my diet so that I would be properly hydrated as water alone is not enough to get the body hydrated. I have taken to eating cucumber which helps and also taking an energade drink every other day just to help get and keep me well hydrated.

I also have to ensure that I drink at least three to four litres of water to be sufficiently hydrated.

My personal survival kit can be broken down easily into the following:

- Faith and reliance in God
- A refusal to accept challenges as proof of finality in any situation.
- Eating healthy and more organic food
- Taking my prescribed medications, the ABC's for SCD: anti-malaria, Folic acid

Multi vitamin supplements (these are vitamin b, c) I also take zinc and cod liver oil supplements for optimal health. I try to eat as much fruit as I can and green vegetables especially those rich in iron like our local sweet potato leaves pumpkin leaves and cassava leaves.

I also try to keep active by walking around a lot and engaging in light exercises such as stretching and some push-ups, nothing overly vigorous.

Being mentally strong and keeping warm or cool depending on weather conditions as well as maintaining good hydration.

Also, am currently taking hydroxy urea. My HB has tended to be my biggest problem in living with SCD. So, in addition to juicing and eating more greens, I was also placed on hydroxy urea very recently.

In conclusion, living with Sickle cell Anaemia is a battle, a daily one, it is not easy, it is not a battle of one's choosing, it is simply thrust upon a person from birth. However, as with any other chronic condition, it is manageable and does not spell only gloom for the affected person SCD brings with it a lot of challenges, but life is always worth living when one finds and gives purpose to their existence. You will always find that a person living with SCD understands pain, knows how to handle it themselves and after the crisis is done or even when it has briefly eased off returns to smiles and laughter as if they had been in such agony before. I have come to learn that in life, no one owes anyone anything except a helping hand when they are able and that anyone can live through anything with God by their side. I have also learnt that no one of us knows our future except God but we can be sure of this, with Him in our lives we can achieve much and get through much and ultimately live very fulfilling rewarding and healthy lives.

I hold to this promise daily: "Surely goodness and mercy shall follow me all the days of my life and I shall dwell in the house of The Lord forever". Psalms 23v 6 and

My motto:" I will surely see the goodness of The Lord in the land of the living " Psalms 27:13.

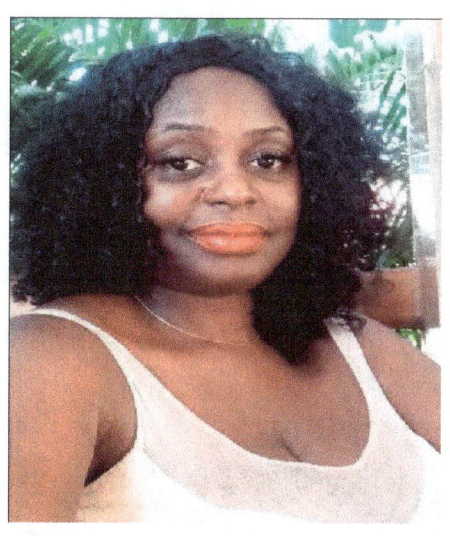

Sickle Cell: A Journey of Hope and Strength
By Mngure Daisy

I was born 43 years ago by both Nurses; my mother is a Nurse Midwife, and my father was a Nurse Anaesthetist. My parents are both Haemoglobin AS. I have 5 siblings. 2 of us are Haemoglobin SS. My father is late.

As a growing child, I didn't have many challenges with Sickle Cell Disease until I left home to be in a boarding school at 12 years. Every now and then, I was brought home from school because of one sickle cell crisis or the other, my parents always nursed me to recovery since both were nurses. L left secondary school in 1997.

I had a real and serious challenge with sickle cell while I was in the university. I was schooling in another state far from my parents and home. Feeding and upkeep became difficult because they had other children to pay school fees, feed and clothe. By this time, none of my parents were working formally, they had worked for mostly missionary establishments and voluntarily retired, then established their private practice but it wasn't doing well.

While in the university, I met a man with whom I became pregnant. I cohabited with him throughout the gestation period. At a point, I became depressed because it looked like I was jumping from frying pan to fire, as the man was not well to do and couldn't even afford the basic antenatal routine drugs a pregnant woman needed. I went through the pregnancy not taking my routine drugs as I seemed quite strong. I birthed the child; a daughter and after the rigours of childbirth I couldn't even get a beverage to refresh myself. A few hours later, I went into a severe crisis. The crisis was so serious that I had to be put on oxygen to enable me to breathe. A few weeks after I was stabilized, I couldn't walk or sit properly because of pains in the hip.

I was diagnosed with avascular necrosis of (R) head of femur. My bills in the hospital were taken care of by a certain tribal woman who came from the same hometown as my parents. She signed that her salary would be used to offset my hospital bills. She was working in the same hospital I gave birth. Because of ill health, my parents were called upon to come and take care of me. My parents came over to the state where I was schooling and where I gave birth as my caregivers. By this time, the man I had the child with was nowhere to be found, and to date, he has not been responsible for the school fees of the daughter she sired or her upkeep.

My parents took me back home with my daughter, the man I had the child with was nowhere to be found. My parents were forced to handle the extra responsibility. I started looking for a remedy to avascular necrosis with limited knowledge of what it was. By this time, I had earlier voluntarily withdrawn from the university for a session, due to the embarrassment of being pregnant out of wedlock and to avoid being stressed since pregnancy is also a stressor to those living with sickle cell. The withdrawal availed me the opportunity to recuperate and take care of my infant.

The pains from the avascular necrosis increased and I had to use a walking cane to ambulate well. I returned to school after 9 months and graduated in a period of 2 years with a 2:2 and a degree in Food Science and Technology. After many hospital visitations, I was booked for hemiarthroplasty, (a partial hip replacement surgery) where the necrosed bone was to be cut and replaced with an implant. I underwent the surgery but couldn't walk months after on my own because the implant used was obsolete and wrongly fixed.

The ability to sit without the implant practically touching my flesh was impossible so I continued walking using crutches as an aid for mobility. 6 months after, I reported to the clinic complaining bitterly and an X-ray was carried out and it was clearly seen the implant had pulled out from the socket of the acetabulum and was loosely hanging thereby touching my flesh. I was there and then, that another surgery was recommended. The second surgery was carried out but there were still no commendable results. I still couldn't walk on my own, the implant used was still the obsolete one (Austin-Moore) and was fixed right into the acetabulum not allowing me the flexibility to ambulate the joint. The Orthopaedic Dr who did the surgery advised I should seek a second opinion for total hip surgery. I refused angrily and continued using a walking stick as support to walk.

Shortly after I got a job, I was elated as I would relieve my parents of the burden of taking care of myself and my daughter. When I started work, it became difficult walking about with the walking aid and also taking care of my daughter, although I had help at home. One day, I couldn't walk again because of the pain and was placed on bed rest. I knew the time for the "second opinion" was knocking. Because I just started work and I couldn't afford the money for the Total Hip Replacement Surgery. A GoFundMe account was opened on my behalf and friends, family and friends of friends rallied around me to raise money for the surgery, which was about #1,400.000M (3115.158 US Dollars). I sought other opinions but this time around from core orthopaedic hospitals and settled for one that had a track record of success in almost all their orthopaedic surgeries done at the facility. I had the surgery done in 2016 and it was successful, and I have had no cause to complain of anything to date.

My name is Mngure, Daisy Mngu. A single parent to an adorable 16-year-old daughter.
I am a Sickle Cell Survivor.

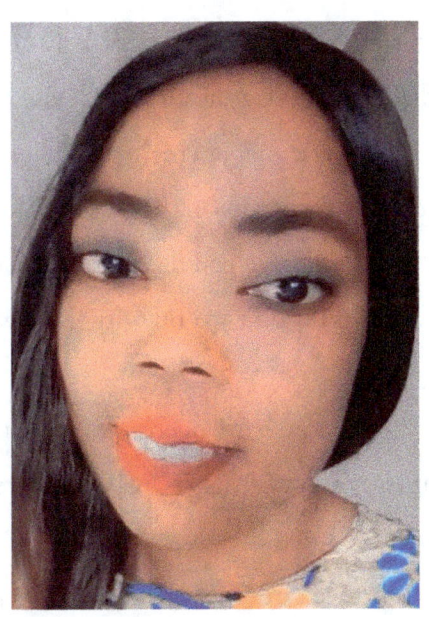

How Sickle Cell Has Impacted Me
By Patricia Chileshe

I am a mother of a 4 year old son who was born with sickle cell. During this period, from the time he was born, I have been having a lot of challenges with him. It's in and out of hospital because of this same condition. When he was born, his health looked to be normal until he started growing up that's when he started showing some symptoms like joint pain, chest pains pale skin and shortness of breath. When we took him to the hospital that's when they diagnosed him as sickle cell anemia.

From that time his health was not okay. He started going to pre-school but because of his health challenges, he ended up stopping cause of so many crises which later on affected his left hand and leg too.

When he stopped going to school, he needed much attention and care. This really affected me as a mother. I used to work because of pains and many crises, the management decided to terminate my contract. So, I had to concentrate on my sickle cell child. That's how I lost my job cause of the sickle cell disease. This came with a lot of challenges of how to find money to buy drugs and how to maintain his diet as well.

Currently, am unable to do what I need to do because I spend most of my time monitoring him. That has really affected my life too. I have to take him for medical examinations, and he has been hospitalized a lot. These are the challenges I am dealing with, sometimes I cry. I have to talk to people to explain my emotions. I talk to family members who have understood and accepted the challenge I have as a mother.

The condition of my child has brought a lot of emotions and strains on my family. There are many interpersonal relationships within the family. Even the family environment has been affected. Because of this sickness. I am unable to participate in social activities outside of our family.

The other factor is that I have no social support from any family members other than my mom, who is also hypertension.

The other impact of sickle cell on me is psychosocial stress. I have been badly stressed with my child's sickness. The demands of caring for my sick child and the feeling of powerlessness over my child's illness caused emotional stress and I became vulnerable.

In addition to the stress, am struggling with depression and anxiety. When my child is in a pain crisis and seeing him lying on the bed at the hospital, it really kills me and I think a lot. This puts me in deep thoughts that I don't see anything to be good and I get depressed. Have gone through psychosocial, physical and financial burdens, because of my sick child, I have realized that, it is important to enhance awareness of this disease by increasing the knowledge of parents and caregivers about SCD.

Education programs are required to enhance mother's awareness about self-care and taking care of our ill children. Awareness among close family members, relatives, friends and the community would also be extremely helpful for social support. Financial support is required to lessen our stress.

Besides this financial support, I feel a multidisciplinary approach to managing the disease and psychosocial support is required for the management of sickle cell and to minimize the burden on both patients and families, I feel it is important to improve the psychosocial problems faced by the patients, caregivers and family members. Lack of knowledge of the causes of disease and its treatment, along with social, cultural and religious factors, adds to the psychosocial burden. Therefore, the efficient therapeutic intervention of SCD requires an all-inclusive scientific understanding, interpretation and perception regarding sickle cell. Long-term psychosocial support is required to help reduce emotional distress, improve compliance with treatment and strengthen coping strategies to improve the quality of life for sickle cell patients and their family members.

Mothers and caregivers must be supported through appropriate counselling programs and enhancing self-care knowledge. I also feel that holistic nursing interventions can support parents and motivate us to cope with our psychosocial and physical burdens. A good example of such intervention is arranging programs to educate parents about taking care of their sick children. So by doing this, the knowledge regarding the disease by healthcare professionals through regular educational programs would help mothers and caregivers reduce their psychosocial problems.

Emphasis must be given to prevention by performing screening tests and antenatal diagnosis. This will play a great role in preventing the disease. Genetic counselling will allow the parents to have a better understanding of the nature of the disease, its consequences, transmission, risks and ways of prevention of transmission and thus parents can make the right decision regarding the ways of prevention if any.

Lack of knowledge, ignorance of the disease and lack of premarital screening practices, I feel it plays a major role in the propagation of this disease. Sickle cell caregivers are mostly unaware of the disease condition that actually acts as the source of sickle cell. Only premarital screening can detect this condition. However, many people would be reluctant or afraid to do the screening tests due to social norms and its adverse effect on their marriage prospects or due to ignorance about the disease.

Being the mother of a sickle cell child, there could be many times I could see and feel that I have failed to look and take care of my child. I, therefore, suggest the following tips for parenting a child with sickle cell:

Be Attentive.

Pay keen attention to things people in your circles say about your child. Everyone is a suspect when it comes to verbal abuse and bullying of a child with sickle cell. From experience, the people closest to you are abusers.

In addition to attention, parents must protect and support a child. Know their triggers and try your best to help her/ him avoid them or not expose him/her to them.

Try to never mind them or their health condition. They know or they could not know because they are young. Most times, we just want to feel like everyone else has a taste of what it feels like. Mostly to see if we are missing something or if not a big deal. Try to give them that. If a crisis occurs, stay by their side and help them through the pain.

Be Involved.

Find ways to get involved in your child's medical routine. Join your child to take routine medications. Folic acid especially is vital in the lines of sickle cell patients. However, this becomes difficult because it's an everyday routine. To make your child feel better, you can make it compulsory for the entire family to take folic acid every day. This intern encourages your child to take it every day as it's visible to him that you are in this together.

Provide Physical Support.

Physical support goes beyond providing a shoulder to lean on, medication, healthcare and staying by the sick bed.

Be grateful for the people in your life. Let's appreciate the few loved ones whom we have, and do not make us feel responsible for our children's illness. The few ones who are there, even if those crises could be avoided.

Be Your Child's Best Friend.

As a parent, your support is the most important need of your child. Especially when they are facing a challenge like sickle cell. Be your child's best friend. Sickle cell comes with a lot of prejudice from the outside, even from close relatives.

Try to create space and room for your child to lean on you all the time. Be that pillar that never bends when it comes to your child living with sickle cell. If you rebuke your child when the whole world seems to be against them, they may begin to see reasons not to exist. No one wants to live in a world where they feel unwanted. Be that person who assures them that they are enough and needed no matter how tough it gets. Give them a reason to keep moving.

Last but not least, take small steps. Parenting a child with special needs like sickle cell is a handful. Try taking it one step at a time and I am sure you will arrive at a better parenting routine for our children. Also, remember to take care of yourself so you can be fit and healthy enough to be there for your children. They need us.

In conclusion, my life has never been the same as the way I used to be. The sickle cell disease crisis can happen at any time. This is how

(SICKLE CELL DISEASE) has impacted me, it is with full challenges that need serious attention by the mother of the sick child.

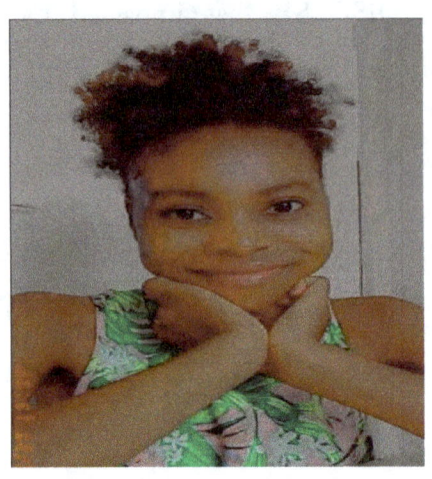

My Sickle Cell Trait Journey
By Phostina Mwansa

Introduction

My name is Phostina Mwansa. I am a Bemba Zambian citizen and live in Lusaka, Zambia. I am 25 years old, and I am a symptomatic sickle cell carrier (AS), I carry a normal gene and an abnormal gene which is the sickle cell trait.

What Is Sickle Cell Trait?

Sickle cell trait (SCT) is not a disease, but having it means that a person has inherited the sickle cell gene from one of his or her parents. With Sickle Cell Trait? People with SCT might experience complications of SCD, such as "pain crises" and, in extreme circumstances, sudden death. More research is needed to find out why some people with SCT have complications and others do not.

In their extreme form and in rare cases, the following conditions could be harmful for people with SCT:
- Increased pressure in the atmosphere (e.g., while scuba diving).
- Low oxygen levels in the air (e.g., when mountain climbing, exercising extremely hard in military,

RENAL MEDULLARY CARCINOMA: This is a type of cancer that affects people with sickle cell trait.

My Childhood Experience

My childhood experiences were quite normal, and I hardly had any health complications not till when I was 11 years in January, I got sick for a year and some months and I was medically ok, I went through a lot, couldn't do anything on my own and almost died. From 2011, my immune system became weak and weaker as I grew older. I was easily affected by different infections during my teenage, my legs could give me severe pain which affected my education and all I was told was that I might have iron deficiency and so I needed to be on iron medication. I wasn't always sick, I could get sick once or twice a month which seemed normal for my family and me.

In 2016, my legs started hurting so badly once again and got worse with the time that I couldn't lift my leg or walk normally, I had prolonged diarrhoea, swollen lips, yellow eyes and now sickle cell came into the picture, ain't sure the tests that were conducted on me but the only thing they found was that I had yeast in stool, got some treatments done and I was alright. My final secondary school exams were a month ahead and so I had to get better as soon as possible.

In April 2020, my body started giving me signs, of excruciating pain and it went on for a month, in May I got flu and was in bed for the whole week, I had never had such flu in my entire life and from then, I never got better.

I started experiencing chest pains after the flu and went to the hospital, I was given some injections and I felt better, after some days, the chest pains were back, my right hand was hurting and could swell up, and I was now having pain in my bones, so I went back to the clinic where I was again given injections to take away the pain which helped for a week and the pain was back again.

I was on and off the medication and pain for the whole month and by then, I lived at my granny's place, I went to mum's house so I could go to some private hospitals to know what was really wrong, as usual, I was told my calcium levels were low hence resulting to bone pains.

I was put on Diclofenac injections again and some calcium tablets, I was also encouraged to take milk more often, etc.

After my injections, I went back to granny's house and was pain-free for a week, the stabbing chest pain came back, including my whole joints hurting this time, so I went back to the clinic and now I was given a transfer to the university teaching hospital.

My Diagnosis

My first appointment there didn't go as well as I expected, I did a chest x-ray to check for Pneumonia and other possible tests, I also noticed a lump on my breast and got it checked for breast cancer, everything came out ok and this time, the doctors didn't know what was wrong with me so I got an appointment to see specialist doctors, specifically specialized in Bones.

My first appointment with a specialist doctor was very good and immediately after I explained all my symptoms, he asked about my health background, according to him I looked younger than my age and all the symptoms were associated with sickle cell, so I did all the tests which showed I have sickle cell trait, because sickle cell trait is said to be benign, the doctors on my next appointments didn't agree with me or with the results of being a carrier and have all sickle cell symptoms, so I was told I have the disease on my other 2 appointments, on my fifth appointment, this time I met two specialists who said I was misdiagnosed and needed to get a Haemoglobin Electrophoresis test done in order to confirm if I have the disease or trait.

The results came in and it showed that 34 % of my cells were sickled and that it was just a trait so I was given another appointment to Haematology.

I had about 5 appointments with different haematologists who believed there's no such a thing as a symptomatic carrier, according to them, sickle cell trait is benign and asymptomatic, and the symptoms and health issues I had didn't mean a thing, so I was discharged from the sickle cell clinic with a prescription of Diclofenac, folic acid and tramadol, the last one said I had to manage to live with it and that the pain is just inside my head and from then never seeing a haematologist again.

Sickle Cell Trait Effect as a Symptomatic Carrier

As a symptomatic carrier, sickle cell trait has caused a drastic turn in my life, I never thought I could get sick and never heal. I am unable to work because of the pain, I lost my job and the conditions aren't favourable for me to work without getting sick. The struggles of doing daily chores without any help, fatigue, insomnia, depression, hardships in keeping relationships and medical/hospital bills.

Being always sick has become my new normal and 24/7 job not because I want it this way but because my body doesn't allow me to do anything without experiencing excruciating pain. Sickle cell trait awareness.

I choose to advocate for myself as a Symptomatic Sickle cell carrier because if I don't, no one else will.

Symptomatic sickle cell carriers live a life full of pain, not only the excruciating pain our body makes us go through but also the pain of not being recognized, not being heard, not having adequate treatment and care. Being told that we exaggerate the pain we go through, whilst it's real.

Going to the hospital to seek medical help and coming back home worse than you went because the doctor thought you were faking the pain and says you are fine and stable.

Being told you just have to manage and live with the pain because there's nothing that can be done by the medical world.

Having to fight medically, emotionally, spiritually, and physically. Being stigmatized and discriminated against just because you are a carrier.

What Does Sickle Cell Trait Pain Feel Like?

It's like a deep, internal pain that you can't escape. It's like your insides are being
ripped apart.
It's like a constant pressure in your lower back that won't go away. It feels like you
are being crushed from the inside out.
It's like a never ending cycle of pain, fatigue, insomnia and frustration. It feels
like your body is betraying you.
It feels like your skin is on fire.
It feels like a deep, stabbing pain that takes your breath away. It's like a constant
dull ache that makes it hard to concentrate.
It feels like you're constantly walking around with heavy weight in your joints. It's
like a sharp shooting pain that comes out of nowhere.
It's like your body is punishing you for something you didn't do. It feels like a
knife is being stubbed in the bones.
It's like fighting your own body which constantly wants to die.

They Said!!

It's just a trait they said, there's absolutely nothing wrong, you will live a normal life. Sickle cell trait is not a disease, you just carry the disease, they said.

You will live a normal life, with no health complications, they said. Sickle cell trait is a benign condition, so whatever pain you say you feel may be

growing pain or it's all in your head, they said.
Only stay hydrated, avoid high altitudes and sky diving, they said.
It's not something to worry about nor do you need any medical plans, they said.
If the growing pain comes back, just take some painkillers and prescribe some
steroids for the growing pain, they said. what they forgot to say was:

not everyone with sickle cell trait is asymptomatic.
there will be times when my Haemoglobin will go low. And I may
be a Symptomatic Sickle cell carrier.
That all the pain crises I go through may be because of the percentage of sickled
cells that I have.
I don't have a normal life, but I always try the best I can to live a life that people
and society will consider normal.
They didn't tell me that the side effects of the pain medicine are so
bad for my health and that the steroid I have been given is very
addictive.
That some days I would wake up tired like I hadn't rested at all.
Fatigue and
insomnia are part of the package.
Nobody told me anything about the mental breakdowns.
In as much as this is just a condition, it is deadly, and the world has recorded a
number of deaths due to sickle cell trait.
They did not tell me that it has its own complications like infection and a high
risk of cancer.
They didn't say a thing about giving up on what I love doing because of my sickle.

cell trait.
No one said a thing about having to advocate for myself and fight to be recognized. No body absolutely nobody told me how to handle all these when.
they come.

My Experience as a Symptomatic Carrier

In my experience, one of the most insidious things about sickle cell trait is that it is an invisible illness.

This means that even though you are a Symptomatic carrier, and your body may be in a constant state of fighting itself, people might not know about your battle just by looking at you.

This is difficult because even if you feel horrible, you might look fine at the same time. In return, people might dismiss your pain and difficulties simply because you don't "look sick".

I have had several vaso occlusive crises that led to hospital admissions, I have had crisis's which lasted for a month and more.

Even being in the hospital is a challenge because not every doctor truly believes you are in pain and so I am always discharged earlier even before I feel better all because I am a carrier.

Mostly, I experience pain in every joint, I also have a hormonal imbalance which causes my ovaries to swell and hurt, I am also losing my eyesight, pain in my ear and I have battled different infections.

I am still learning how to manage all these symptoms and crises, I have adopted an autoimmune diet just to maintain all my symptoms, heat and cold therapy has really helped me manage all my symptoms,

I have also been considerate of my environment, and taking one day at a time.

I now experience some pain-free days and go into remission if I follow the rules and listen to my body.

Stigma and Discrimination

Sickle cell comes with stigma and discrimination, so does the trait. We are in a society where a warrior has to fake being ok, always trying to fit in, act normal or you will be considered cursed, avoided and laughed at all because of how your body looks, how you are always in pain and because of lack of awareness, others think it's contagious and try by all means to avoid contacts.

we don't just fight the pain physically but also socially, taking risks and sometimes ignoring our symptoms all in the name of fitting in because people will look at me weirdly if I were to start limping from nowhere or scream out in desperate pain, stigma has made a lot of symptomatic warriors not to say a thing about the pain they go through because everyone say it's benign not even doctors believe it, lair, attention seeker, deceitful, sympathy seeker is what a carrier is called for opening up to the community and medical world at large for experiencing sickle cell crisis as a carrier. Symptomatic carriers mostly face discrimination in the hospital, as we are treated differently from full-blown warriors despite experiencing the same pain at the same time, many times that I was sent back home, and discharged from the hospital with the same level of pain all because I am a carrier and it's said I must not have any health issues, having symptoms means nothing as long as it's sickle cell trait, it doesn't matter. Negligence is more common in sickle cell trait because we have no care plan, or follow-ups and are never given sufficient treatment.

People will judge you just by the way you look, the way you do things, missing dates, appointments and not always being available.

Because of all these acts, a lot of carriers have died, committed suicide and have mental health breakdowns.

The pain itself can cause depression and it only gets worse with the stigma and discrimination.

It hurts more than a place where we are supposed to find help is the worst place where we get neglected, ignored, misunderstood and zero treatment, people who are supposed to make us feel better are the worst nightmares because they don't believe the pain is there and don't give any treatment, we hardly beg and scream in agony in order to be looked at and given treatment, this breaks me down every time I experience such and become worsens my situation.

Sickle cell trait has also affected me financially, I am an engineer by profession, jobless because I couldn't keep up with my last job, every tiny task caused a painful crisis which made me unreliable and disqualified for the position.

I can't keep a job because there are no precautions for someone like me.

Managing hospital bills and pain medicine has affected my family and me, I can't leave a day without any pain medicine, it is quite expensive I don't cater to it by myself but need help from my family and thank God they come through for all my needs, sometimes I can't help it but think am a burden because crisis come unannounced and I see my family struggle and postponed other things just to make sure I get the treatment and medicine I need.

I face financial challenges because I can't always get what I want but just what I need. There's a very heavy weight that comes with sickle cell trait and financial challenges.

You Are Strong and Brave!

Have you ever asked yourself and weighed the energy and potential that you have for sickle cell trait??

Fighting something which is considered benign medically is not an easy task because for every treatment, you will have to explain yourself over and over again which sometimes they never believe, but just like the widow wanting justice from the judge, I keep persisting and explaining and crying just so I am given something to ease my pain, and every time that am actually believed and attended to, I clap for myself and say " damn I made it, I have actually convinced them" and that's a win for me.

If there's one thing am proud of is the strength I possess towards every crisis and pain. It doesn't matter how long the pain lasts but as long as it goes away and sets me free, it's an achievement because it's never easy fighting your own body.

It's rare to wake up with 0 pain, there's always that pain that won't just go and give you a pain-free day(my right hip and knee are always in pain and so I take my painkillers every day just to maintain and avoid worsening the situation) and that's the " am fine " for me, but that doesn't stop me from doing one or two things, as I wake up every morning just like any other person, I make plans for the day and sometimes I literally get nothing done or out of the 5,6,7 things I had planned to do, if I get 1,2 or 3 things done it's a win for me and am so proud and can happily say I got things done.

If you wake up in the morning with your body giving you signs and any kind of unpleasant feeling/ pain but still you choose to ignore it and do what you've got to do for the day, my fellow warrior you are strong and be proud of yourself.

Despite feeling bent (that's the term I use when am not having a pain-free day) you still dress up and go to work, you get that job done, you don't cut off your meetings or outings with friends, you are brave and when that happens to me I say to myself "am in charge s.c.t doesn't have me but I have it, it doesn't control me but the other way round". Every day is a battle and I win each and every time, in my mind I go like, what kind of enemy is this? Despite losing every single day, it never give up, then I tell myself if the looser doesn't give up what can make me the winner give up???, and that just gains me more and more strength to fight as it comes.

if it comes at an intense speed, I will activate my intense strength and ability to fight and just when it thinks it has me, then boom, double strength is activated at this point, even though I couldn't stand or walk on my own, I will get up and lean on things and walls as I make my way to the bathroom as a Spartan soldier that I am.

People may say I am lazy, all I do is sit around and sleep, that really doesn't matter to me because deep down in my heart, I know am the strongest, bravest and am proud of the warrior that I am, I have battled and won every kind of pain that sickle cell has inflicted on me, never ever let anyone make you feel less of a human being or that you worth nothing at all, if they were to be in your shoes just for a day, they wouldn't make it as far as you have made it.

The pain we warriors go through drains us mentally in all this, one thing I don't do is question my existence, I know am here for a purpose and God is with me all the way, as He gives me strength to overcome and see another day and that gives me the courage to face each and every day as it comes, if am having a painful day and I can do nothing the eyes can see, it's definitely because am busy fighting the unexplainable pain which I was probably not ready for and so I will do it tomorrow, it doesn't matter how many days I postponed my to-do list, what matters is that I get it done whenever I have the chance.

The joy I get when I can finally get to do all the things I couldn't do is unexplainable, so I use it wisely and get everything done at the end of the day am buffed, I must confess that sometimes it never ends up well, it's just like you have opened the pathways for the enemy to attack but still I put a smile on my face for the things I got done, it's a little achievement for me am sure my fellow warriors know what am talking about. Never let sickle cell complications take charge of your life.

Always be happy.
Always know you are a warrior who is; Unique.
Strong.
Brave.
Loved.
Courageous.

Never quitting. Worthy. Distinguished.
and your pain is just part of your story, not your whole story, live life to the fullest.

My Advocacy

I am a sickle cell trait advocate, I started my advocacy journey in 2021, where I run a Facebook page called "sickle cell trait warrior ", where I share all my experiences with sickle cell trait and speak my mind.

I am happy that I know I am not alone neither am I making up the pain in my mind because there are thousands of us who go through challenges because of sickle cell trait.

I don't want the next generation of symptomatic carriers to go through what I've gone through, to feel betrayed by their own bodies or to feel alone.

I advocate for sickle cell trait because I want to make it known that we aren't crazy or exaggerating, making up the pain, etc. Everything we go through is real and sickle cell trait is the culprit.

Alongside sickle cell trait comes many other diagnoses and I believe it's connected. Below is the link to my page

https://www.facebook.com/traitwarrior?mibextid

phostinamwansa@gmail.com.

Finally, Sickle cell trait is not a benign condition, just like Sickle cell, it affects each one of us differently.

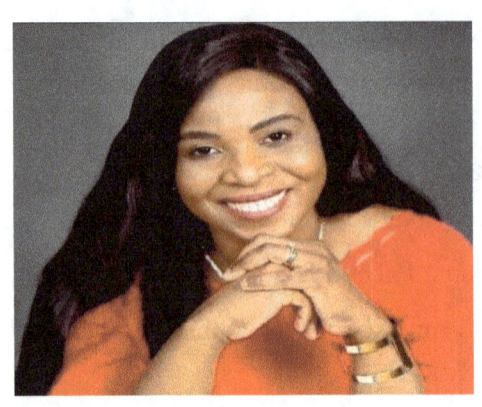

Sickle Cell Disease in Australia and Zambia
A comparison of the two countries I call home.
By Agnes Nsofwa

Introduction

I'm a sickle cell advocate who has dedicated her life to raise awareness about Sickle Cell Disease (SCD) around the world after our daughter was diagnosed at the age of 14 months in the late 2000s. My dedication to this cause was accidental, something that I never anticipated that I would be doing. I'm a shy person, I grew up not having to courage to express myself and was bullied constantly at home and at school. Over the years, I developed the resilience of standing up for myself and in high school I joined in debate team where I could manage different topics with confidence. Being an advocate has challenges, advantages, and disadvantages. I have learned so much since becoming on the scene a few years ago, especially on the global scale. This has somehow made know by different people around the world and this too has been very challenging. I was born in Zambian and migrated to Australia in the early 2000s. Living in two worlds has taught me to appreciate different aspects on life lessons at different levels. Few years after I started my SCD advocacy journey in Australia, I was asked by one of my respected SCD elders to support SCD advocacy in Zambia. Although this been met with a lot of challenges, I still have hope that one day I will create a centre of excellence for sickle cell warriors in Zambia. The key is to never give up. The chapter will elaborate on the differences and similarities between the management of sickle cell disease in Zambia and Australia.

What is Sickle Cell Disease?

The blood disorder known as sickle cell disease (SCD) is caused by inheriting a defective version of the haemoglobin molecule from both parents. Those with SCD have earned the nickname "warriors" for their unyielding spirit in the face of adversity (Kato et al., 2018). The haemoglobin protein in red blood cells is responsible for transporting oxygen across the body. With SCD, the haemoglobin in red blood cells hardens into rods. This causes structural changes in red blood cells. Because of this, the disc-shaped cells transform into crescent or sickle shapes (Brown, 2012).

Sickle-shaped cells are rigid and unable to readily shape-shift. The blood vessels cause a lot of them to disintegrate. Sickle cells only survive 10-20 days, while normal cells live for roughly 90-120 days (Adio et al., 2022). When cells in a patient's body are damaged, it might be difficult for the body to regenerate enough healthy replacement cells. This condition might lead to an insufficiency of red blood cells. A fighter suffering from anaemia may experience extreme fatigue. People with mild sickle cell anaemia/sickle cell trait are resistant to malaria; because the malaria parasites called Plasmodium cannot survive in defective/sickle cell shaped haemoglobin; it has less oxygen concentration. The mutations cause defective sickle cell-shaped haemoglobin. Africa is found in the tropics, which is an endemic malaria area. It is a natural selection in action by Charles Darwin's theory of Natural selection (Kaur et al., 2013). In addition, the sickle-shaped cells may adhere to the vessel walls, blocking blood flow. Because of this, the oxygen supply to adjacent tissues is diminished (Manwani and Frenette, 2013).

How I Knew I'm Impacted By SCD

Over 15 years ago, I was lying in a hospital bed sick with an unknown disease. The doctors were puzzled that they could not understand why my haemoglobin kept dropping by the day, why I had so many white blood cells which was an indication that I had an infection, but numerous blood cultures could not determine what infection I had. I was in excruciating pain and had the worst sore throat.

Unbeknown to the doctors, I was experiencing an acute episode of a condition called Sickle Cell Disease. But what was puzzling was that I'm not a sickle cell disease patient, I simply carry a recessive gene, or I have a sickle cell trait. And I was 7 months pregnant at the time. For 8 weeks, I was admitted to the women's hospital in Perth until doctors decided to use steroids to manage my bizarre symptoms which thanks to the higher being worked and I was induced to give birth to a "healthy" baby at full term. What followed this is the theme for my story today. 12 months after our daughter was born, she was eventually diagnosed with sickle cell disease after numerous signs and symptoms.

The first four years after her diagnosis, my life literally turned upside down. I went through different stages of grief, from self-blame, denial, anger, depression and finally accepting the situation. I blamed myself for not being smart enough to understand our family health history, I further went on bizarre theories that maybe it was a misdiagnosis and that she would eventually get better. Anger kicked in because the hospital system failed us when I had all the signs and symptoms during pregnancy, but they did not act upon that information. You see, had they acted upon the fact that I have the sickle cell gene, they would have tested my husband to find out if he had the gene too. Then, they would have tested our daughter and taken necessary precautions to ensure that they reduced the risks of the symptoms and surgeries she endured before getting a final diagnosis. So, I was angry and almost sued the hospital for negligence. But with hospital appointments every two weeks or so, there was no time for me to go through that path. Instead, I slowly started the healing process.

The process of acceptance involved me telling all our family and friends what our daughter was going through. I also decided to be vocal about this condition, and I later found out that it was a rare disease in Australia. A rare disease is defined as a disease affecting less than 2,000 people in any country. I started off researching as much information as I could about Sickle Cell Disease, I started an online support group at the same time, and I went back to university and enrolled in nursing school.

Four years after I graduated from nursing school, I started a not-for-profit organisation solely supporting people impacted by Sickle Cell Disease in Australia. Since its inception, the Australian Sickle Cell Advocacy Inc (ASCA) has achieved various milestones in the sickle cell community in Australia. One of the notable achievements was creating a sickle cell disease course for healthcare professionals to educate them on the best practices for caring for patients with sickle cell disease. Our organization has also represented Australia at different conferences worldwide and advocated for the expansion of curative therapies for people living with sickle cell disease in Australia. ASCA also organised the first-ever sickle cell conference in Australia which included both the Health Minister and Shadow Minister as guest speakers in September 2021.

After starting a not-for-profit organisation, it dwelt to me, this was my calling. I looked back at the challenging period in our lives and finally found a purpose while caring for my daughter battling sickle cell disease. I never stopped advocating for our daughter. As my organisation was thriving, I was also discussing with doctors to try curing her via the only successful curative option now, a bone marrow transplant. After waiting for almost 10 years due to different circumstances including death in our community by a family member dying after they attempted to do a bone marrow transplant, our daughter was cured from Sickle Cell Disease becoming the first child to be cured of this condition in Australia. This gave me hope and was ready to encourage others around the world.

In the year 2020, I founded Amplify Sickle Cell Voices International Inc (ASVI), a global initiative that empowers sickle cell warriors, caregivers, and advocates to use their voices to change the sickle cell disease narrative. Through this initiative, my main aim is to amplify the voices of those impacted by sickle cell disease to create a better world for them. ASVI is a global movement comprising any person impacted by sickle cell disease either as a patient, caregiver, advocate, healthcare professional, or any well-wish. Furthermore, I co-founded a not-for-profit organization in Zambia my country of origin. Zambian Network for Sickle Cell -Amplified Voices and Advocacy (ZNSAVA) is aimed at raising awareness, education, and support for people impacted by sickle cell disease. As an Executive Director of the ZNSAVA, I work tirelessly to change the sickle cell disease narrative in this country, and our efforts have been instrumental in providing a voice for sickle cell warriors, caregivers, and healthcare providers. Although challenging at times, I have hope that one day sickle cell disease will be considered a public health concern to our policymakers. ZNSAVA is a national organisation whose main aim is to change the sickle cell narratives in all parts of Zambia, especially remote areas. Sickle cell disease predominantly affects people from Sub-Saharan Africa, where Zambia is situated.

Zambia is situated on a high plateau in south-central Africa and takes its name from the Zambezi River, which drains all but a small northern part of the country. It is a landlocked country in Africa with an estimated population of 19.8 million people as of 2022.

Australia is the smallest continent and one of the largest countries on Earth, lying between the Pacific and Indian oceans in the Southern Hemisphere. Australia is the sixth-largest country by land mass, its population is comparatively small with most people living around the eastern and south-eastern coastlines and estimated at 26 million as of 2023.

In terms of Gross domestic product (GDP), there is a huge difference between these two countries. GDP is a monetary measure of the market value of all the final goods and services produced and sold at a specific time by a country or countries.

GDP is most often used by the government of a single country to measure its economic health. According to the IMF, Australia is set to become the world's 12th largest economy in 2023, with a nominal GDP of around A$2.5 trillion (US$1.8 trillion). According to World Economics, Zambia's GDP is estimated to be $109 billion - 68% larger than official estimates.

This picture will help us understand why there are differences in the management of sickle cell disease in these two countries.

In Australia, SCD is considered a rare disease. A rare disease is described as a condition that affects less than 2,000 people in a country. The low prevalence of sickle cell disease in Australia means that few people are familiar with it. The Haemoglobinopathy Registry is tracking the incidence of Sickle Cell Disease in Australia at Monash University's Department of Public Health and Preventive Medicine.

Other than this, only limited secondary research is present to examine different factors associated with sickle cell disease prevalence in Australia and Zambia. Also, little research is present to compare these two countries that highlight the similarities and differences, this will contribute to providing different insights and practices of sickle cell disease in both Zambia and Australia based on the screening tools, interventions, prevalence, and different factors that do have an impact in causing its emergence.

Sickle Cell Disease in Zambia

Sickle Cell Disease (SCD) is the most common genetic condition in Zambia. This disease was previously seen as a low priority in public health due to a lack of research on this crucial subject. In 2017, the University Teaching Hospital in Lusaka saw almost 6,000 new patients in the haematology clinic, becoming highest cases of patients to be treated at this hospital (Sinkala, 2017). Among the clinical signs are recurrent acute and incapacitating pain crises and potentially lethal consequences on the respiratory, heart, kidneys, and nervous systems. Sickle cell illness has evolved as a defense against malaria, which explains why it is so common in several African nations in the tropical regions where malaria is prevalent. Zambia, for example, has one of the worst malaria death tolls among the world's twenty most populous nations. Zambia is home to around 2% of the world's sickle cell disease patients and 5% of the region's cases (Kumar et al., 2014) Shockingly, the incidence of sickle cell began to rise in Zambia in 2020, despite substantial efforts being achieved in the 2010s to suppress the sickness. It turns out that the number of sickle cell cases, testing positives, and deaths rose by 30% to 50% between 2018 and 2019 and again during the first half of 2020 (Simwangala et al., 2022). As there is no information on the frequency or incidence of sickle cell disease in Zambia, we cannot speculate on its effects (Kumar et al., 2014). If the sickle cell trait occurs at a rate of 18 percent, as Barclay discovered in Kitwe, and if there are 246 cases of sickle cell anaemia for every 60,000 individuals, then Zambia, a country of 13 million, would have 63,300 cases of sickle cell anaemia (Siachisa, 2020).

Sickle cell disease affects a substantial percentage of the population in Zambia but has gotten little attention there. With 20-25% of the population carrying the sickle cell trait and 1%-2% of infants born with the ailment (Nwanonyiri, 2018), according to Kings Health Partners.Org, Zambia's Ministry of Health has acknowledged sickle cell disease as a public health hazard (2021). More than sixteen thousand people with sickle cell disease are now registered at the University Teaching Hospitals (UTH) or the Arthur Davison Children's (ADH) haematology clinics. Many kids are here, most of whom are under 15 years old. More than 10% of admissions to Arthur Davison Children's Hospital are due to SCD, making it the leading reason for admission at Children's Hospital-UTH (Simuyaba, 2019).

The data from these medical centres in two distinct locations indicate that sickle cell disease is a significant public health issue that requires immediate attention on a national basis. There are a lot of kids here, most less than 15 years old (15). Many of these people are not diagnosed. Thus, they do not get adequate treatment, if any at all.

Sickle Cell Disease in Australia

Although it is estimated that Sickle Cell Disease (SCD) occurs in about 200 – 1000 per 100,000 births in the developing countries in sub-Sahara Africa and Asia, this condition is considered a rare disease in Australia. A rare disease is defined a condition with a population prevalence of less than 1 in 2000 people in a country. Crighton et al. (2016) indicates that, as Australia becomes increasingly ethnically diverse, the prevalence of SCD will increase due to migration patterns. According to the SCD experts in Australia, sickle cell incidences had increased tenfold in the last 15 years.

Furthermore, haematologists in Australia have observed that SCD disproportionately affects migrant families with socio-economic challenges. A lot of our members from Australian Sickle Cell Advocacy Inc (ASCA), still have challenges to explain SCD to healthcare professionals. It is still common for some nurses or doctors to treat a patient with SCD for the first time. The lack of knowledge and constant explanations of what SCD is, not only to healthcare professionals but the community at large is what prompted me to start ASCA. ASCA was formed due to the frustrations of most families who had to help nurses or doctors understand SCD. What initially started off as an online support group, it was formally registered in 2018.

The vision of ASCA is to reduce the impact of SCD on all affected Australians. ASCA provides a range of highly valued support services including comprehensive patient information as well as emotional and practical support. Since its inception in 2018, the SCD narratives have changed for the better in terms of recognition and knowledge among different stakeholders. ASCA has managed to engage policymakers from the highest health minister's office ensuring that in 2019 for example, SCD impacted families were formally recognised for the first time ever in the Australian history. ASCA continue to fight for change of policies to enhance SCD awareness Australia wide.

The prevalence of SCD cases in Australia is not well known due to the inconclusive numbers captured at the only haemoglobinopathy registry based in Melbourne Australia. According to the staff at this registry, the Registry collects data on thalassaemia and sickle cell disease in adults and children at participating sites across Australia. The data collection is undertaken by clinicians and trained healthcare staff at participating hospitals and data management and analysis is undertaken by Monash University. An opt-off consent model is used at this registry where patients are invited to participate and provided with information about the registry and how to opt-off if the wish.

Data is collected from these sites looking at these variables:

- Demographics
- Diagnosis and testing
- Transfusion therapy (including age at first transfusion, type of transfusion e.g., exchange, and the interval between transfusions)
- Medications and hospital presentations

- Complications of condition or therapy (including VOC))

As of 2019, the registry had 8 sites collecting data and 5 sites had ethics approval but had not contributed to the registry. One of the major challenges for these sites is the lack of funding, making it difficult for sites to allocate staff time for data entry.

In terms of management SCD, warriors are lucky to access free healthcare if you are a permanent resident, citizen or hold a humanitarian visa. The Australian health system is one of the best in the world which is predominantly funded by taxpayers. For us as a family, we were lucky that our daughter's Bone Marrow Transplant (BMT) was funded through this healthcare system. Even though we hold private health insurance and opted to support the hospital to go in as private patients, in an incidence that we did not have this insurance, our daughter was still going to be treated for free.

SCD is mainly managed using hydroxyurea and the only disease modifying drug like most countries, especially in developing countries. If hydroxyurea fails, like in the case of our daughter, then the next option will be blood transfusions or red cell exchange. BMT will be the last option in very few cases. Other medications available in other parts of the world like the USA or Europe are not available yet in Australia.

As we strive to raise awareness about SCD in Australia, I'm proud to be managing ASCA to enhance this objective. ASCA has put SCD in Australia on the map and as of 2023, it will be hosting the 3rd Sickle Cell Scientific Conference. In Australia, some of the different types of SCD include sickle B thalassemia, sickle haemoglobin C disease and sickle cell anaemia (SS disease) (Kazankov et al., 2016).

Australia has introduced different interventions and programs to deal with the severity of this health issue that requires urgent treatment and discussion with a haematology consultant. Sickle cell crisis management has improved in recent years that usually requires detailed assessment by the healthcare expert, including history, examination, and investigation of the patients (Oudin Doglioni et al., 2021). This includes taking a medical history of the patients at risk of having this issue along with their usual treatment. After that, the examination includes the analysis of different symptoms associated with the patients, followed by investigations to find out the main cause of anaemia and to incorporate a treatment intervention (Crighton et al., 2016). I'm very optimistic with the future of SCD awareness in Australia going forward. As an organisation, ASCA is always improving ways and means to increase the awareness countrywide.

Similarities Between Australia and Zambia

Zambia accounts for around 5% of all sickle cell disease cases in eastern and southern Africa and 2% of all cases globally. Due to its rarity, sickle cell disease is mostly unknown in Australia. Only after similarities are present between the equivalence of sickle cell anaemia within Zambia and Australia do some similarities exist between these nations (Liyoka et al., 2022). They have incorporated multiple screening and monitoring tools to include the emergence of this healthcare issue. These nations have also incorporated supported groups within their healthcare institutes to provide the community with effective healthcare services (White et al., 2020). Other than this, for one, in both these countries, children are the ones who are highly impacted by sickle cell disease. This age group suffers greatly from anaemia. One of the contributing reasons why the community within both these nations suffers from sickle cell anaemia is iron deficiency and other hereditary and genetic factors (Musowoya et al., 2020).

The specific management intervention followed by the healthcare communities of both Australia and Zambia is also similar. These nations are using similar general management techniques that include effective monitoring and screening to control the prevalence of sickle cell anaemia (Simuyaba, 2019). The use of hydroxyurea, blood transfusions and red cell exchange, is also common between both countries.

Differences Between Australia and Zambia

Around 2% of all sickle cell disease cases worldwide and 5% in eastern and southern Africa cases are found in Zambia. Sickle cell illness is quite uncommon. Thus, most Australians are unfamiliar with it.

The differences between sickle cell anaemia within Zambia and Australia appear in terms of prevalence and different strategies to control its prevalence. In Zambia, sickle cell anaemia is recognized as a highly prevalent public health problem, per the Zambian Ministry of Health. Also, about 20 to 25% of the population had been suffering from this issue, among which 1 to

2% are newborn babies. On record, the university chief teaching hospitals in Zambia had about 16,000 active sickle cell patients on a record. Besides this, most of the age at which sickle cell anaemia is prevalent is under 15 years (Simwangala et al., 2022; Simuyaba, 2019). The increased prevalence of sickle cell disease in Zambia has been causing biochemical abnormalities and pathological consequences in patients. It also leads to cause serious disease issues within the individuals (Kahindo et al., 2022). In 2019, Zambia still faced the increased diagnosis of sickle cell in India. The World Health Organization has also dictated that this is one of the major issues within Africa, including Zambia. Also, most children below the age of five usually die due to the severity of anaemia. To address this healthcare issue, Zambia has also introduced different screening programs to deal with this issue. The Zambia screening program will screen 10,000 newborn babies by developing an electronic database including laboratory records, history, and patient demographics. It includes screening the babies at three different sites to ensure diagnosis and treatment of this issue (Makoni, 2021; Muzazu et al., 2022).

Some of the causes associated with the prevalence of sickle cell disease within Africa from last Zambia include lack of health ministries and their involvement. In most of their cases, this healthcare issue is also caused by the homozygosity for "β-globin S gene mutation (SS disease)." (Suali et al., 2023). Other than this, the social factor that is associated with enhancing its prevalence is the lack of high-intensity medical care and the limited excess of the community towards it. These are some of the reasons that are associated with causing sickle cell disease within Zambia (Liyoka et al., 2022).

However, in contrast, Australia has a rare prevalence of sickle cell disease, so most of the community is unaware of this healthcare issue. Although experts predict that there are about 1,000 incidences of SCD in Australia, the exact data is not available. But still, sickle cell anaemia in Australia is prevalent due to increased immigration. It is one of the social and cultural factors associated with its prevalence (Ellis et al., 2022). The increased ethical diversity enhanced the prevalence of haemoglobin-related disorders, including sickle cell disorder and thalassemia.

The statistics of sickle cell anaemia within Australia include 12% of the women suffering from this issue, and about 8% of preschool-aged children have SCD. Other than this, about 20% of individuals over 85 years are anaemic. Overall, it has been estimated that about 1.1 million Australians are iron deficient, one of the major contributing factors to sickle cell disease (Greenway et al., 2022). The Australian Healthcare System and Health Ministries are effective enough in controlling this healthcare issue. The Australian healthcare sector has incorporated multiple interventions and healthcare experts to treat sickle cell disease patients. The children who suffer from this healthcare issue require immediate hospitalization to deal with any complications. Although the Australian healthcare system does not have the Newborn Screening for SCD program in place yet, the public health system has timely management of vaso-occlusive crisis and other protocols for controlling this disease (Eithier et al., 2020). Hematopoietic stem cell transplantation (HSCT) is currently the only established curative intervention for SCD that can restore normal haematopoiesis. (Kanter et al., 2021). In Australia, this curative option started in 2019, and my daughter was the first child to undergo this treatment. Since then, there have been about 5 children as of 2023, who have undergone this treatment. This therapy requires one to have a sibling donor to have a higher success rate. Hence most of these procedures conducted in Australia have required a sibling donor.

The treatment option also required extensive testing beginning with a Human leukocyte antigen (HLA) a genetic test used to match patients and donors for bone marrow, cord blood, or organ transplants. All these tests including the actual curative therapy are free for Australian Citizens, Permanent Residents, and those on special visas. Aftercare is also very extensive with outpatient hospital appointments scheduled vigorously for 12 months post the procedure.

On the other hand, the Zambian health system does not offer this curative therapy. Even though we have a lot of people living with sickle cell disease, the healthcare system coupled with living standards in this developing country has made it impossible for most patients to benefit from this treatment option. What tends to happen is that most families will opt to take their children if they can afford it. The Zambian government does not support 100% of fees and only a few families are supported with minimal contribution towards this treatment. As a result, the most effective means for most Zambian sickle cell patients is to manage living with SCD in a meaningful healthy way to avoid symptoms and complications to avoid organ damage or mental health issues affecting the physical healing and SCD management.

In terms of Advocacy, there are three organisations that work to raise awareness about SCD in Australia. Two organisations which are predominantly Thalassaemia organisations do some work to do SCD awareness. Australian Sickle Cell Advocacy Inc is the only organisation created to raise awareness about sickle cell disease in Australia. It serves as a support advocacy group that has provided the community with basic rights and awareness to navigate the healthcare system in Australia.

In contrast, In Zambia, there are numerous patient organisations with most of them based in Lusaka Zambia, the country's capital. Organisations are different in nature consisting of charity organisations, individuals and Doctors all advocating for sickle cell awareness.

To summarize, the differences between sickle cell disease in Zambia and Australia are in the prevalence, screening, and monitoring tests. Other than this, different cultural and socioeconomic sector factors are associated with the prevalence of this healthcare issue within these two countries. Sickle cell disease is more prevalent within Zambia as compared to Australia.

While Australia has the facilities to perform curative therapy of bone marrow transplant to cure SCD, Zambia is still far off from having such facilities and will depend on countries like India to have their citizens cured of SCD. Australia has one main organisation to raise awareness about SCD while Zambia has several organisations with most of them based in Lusaka Zambia.

Room For Improvement for SCD in Zambia

The only treatment for SCD is a bone marrow transplant or stem cell transplant. The donors and recipients must be very similar for a bone marrow transplant to be effective. Some of the finest organ donors are brothers and sisters. As a result, only a select few Zambian households can afford to have this treatment option. Anyone in Zambia needing this therapy must go to other nations, such as India, to get it (Salinas Ciseros and Thein, 2020).

Antibiotics, such as penicillin, that prevent bacterial infections in children under the age of 5 are recommended by Zambia's national SCD guidelines and may help with symptom alleviation, problem reduction, and life extension (Ballas, 2020).

Various pain relievers, including morphine, ibuprofen, diclofenac, and paracetamol, are used in severe instances. If you or someone you know has SCD and is experiencing a pain crisis, they can assist (Herity et al., 2021).

Hydroxyurea is effective in treating and preventing a variety of SCD symptoms. Anaemia has been alleviated, thanks to the rise in fetal haemoglobin levels that this supplement causes. Even though this medication is vital for SCD patients, most parents cannot afford to purchase it regularly due to the limited availability of this treatment via government agencies. When taken daily, hydroxyurea reduces the frequency of painful crises and might reduce the need for blood transfusions and hospitalizations (Lattanzi et al., 2021).

Patients with sickle cell disease do not have a balanced ratio of nitric oxide within their blood. This is one of the major reasons why blood vessels get blocked. Therefore, it is recommended that the patients need to be provided with nitric oxide to provide room for improving sickle cell disorder (Matte et al., 2019).

The usage of ultrasound machines like transcranial will help in the measurement of blood flow within sickle cell disease. This will contribute to dictating the possibility of having stroke risk and controlling its prevalence. It will also enhance awareness among healthcare experts regarding using regular blood transfusion to control stroke (Henry et al., 2021).

Recommendations

- Have a healthy, well-rounded diet and take folic acid supplements regularly. New red blood cells are made in the bone marrow with the help of vitamins like folic acid. See your physician for questions about folic acid or other vitamin supplements. Fruits, vegetables, and whole grains should all be staples in your diet (Neumayr et al., 2019).

- Keep your body hydrated by drinking plenty of water. It is more probable that you will have a sickle cell crisis if you are dehydrated. Aim for eight 8-ounce glasses of water daily. Drink more water if you are engaging in strenuous activity or if you will be spending time in a hot, dry area (Ali et al., 2020).

- Stay away from temperature extremes. Extreme temperatures or humidity might trigger a sickle cell crisis (Minniti et al., 2021).
- Try to maintain a regular exercise routine without overdoing it. See your doctor if you want to know how much exercise is safe for you.
- It would be best to exercise caution while using any drug you buy without a prescription. It is recommended that pain relievers containing ibuprofen or naproxen sodium (Aleve) be used cautiously, if at all, due to the risk of kidney impairment. Consult your doctor before using any OTC medication (Darbari et al., 2020).
- Don't light up. Having a severe pain episode is more likely if you smoke.
- It is recommended that patients with SCD need focus on nutritional considerations to address this issue. These include:

1. High-calorie, nutrient-dense diet
2. Maintain hydration.
3. "Supplementation of zinc, magnesium, and vitamins A, C, and E or treatment with high-dose antioxidants can reduce the percentage of irreversibly sickled.
4. cells."
5. Including omega 3, supplemental EPA, and DHA help reduce severe anaemia (Farooq and Testai, 2019).

- Zambia needs to focus on controlling the prevalence of sickle cell disease by increasing the effectiveness of screening and monitoring strategies. The effective execution of the screening will contribute to dealing with this crisis (Matte et al., 2019).

- Australia needs to increase awareness within the community regarding this healthcare due to its rarity, especially in different multicultural communities.

Conclusion

Sickle cell disease (SCD) is a group of inherited disorders caused by mutation on the haemoglobin α or/and β- chain, which includes sickle cell anaemia and thalassemia. Mutation of this kind obstructs the biological function of blood haemoglobin. About 300,000 infants are born with SCD globally, and it is estimated that sickle cell anaemia occurs in about 200 – 1000 per 100,000 births in the developing countries in sub-Sahara Africa and Asia (1,2). Crighton et al.

While SCD is rare in Australia, relatively few locals have heard of it. Despite the high prevalence of sickle cell disease in Zambia, the country has paid little attention to it. According to Kings Health Partners.Org, 1–2% of newborns in Zambia have sickle cell disease. This has led to the Zambian Ministry of Health classifying sickle cell disease as a public health risk (2021). Examining sickle cell disorder within both countries has also suggested that it is significantly highly prevalent within Zambia because of different socioeconomic and cultural factors. Besides this, the health ministry system efficiency and screening and monitoring are also highly effective within Australia compared to Zambia.

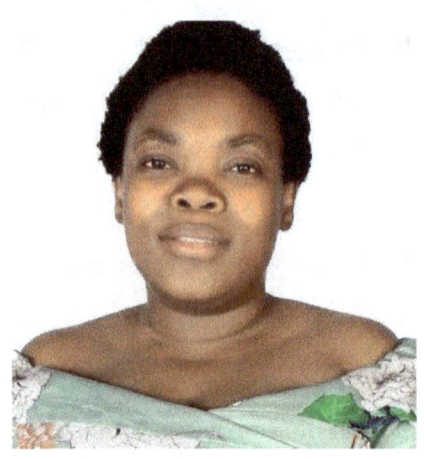

The comparison of Sickle Cell Care between Uganda and the United Kingdom
By Solome Mealin

My name is Solome Mealin (Nee Nanziri); I was born and raised in Uganda, born in a village called Kitovu, in Masaka District; but I was raised in Konge sub-parish, Makindye division, Kampala district and Ntinda before I came to the United Kingdom.

I was diagnosed with sickle cell disease when I was four years old. I used to get so sickly and cried a lot as a baby, but no one knew why I was like that. One day, when I was four years old, I woke up covered in pain all over my body. I had turned yellow, with no energy and just crying. My Grandma was so shocked as my eyes were all yellow for the first time. She did not know what to do because that time, she had no idea that I had sickle cell disease. She asked her friends around the village, and everyone told her of some herbs that could help. There was these nice elderly man who took it upon himself to get me local herbs every two days for steaming me, washing me with and drinking, and he never asked for money. In Africa, "it takes the entire village to raise a child". That man, I will call him Mr N, was the true example of that quote. He never asked for money or anything. Grandma appreciated him so much and every time she harvested food, she would send him some in the basket.

Another elder who was a doctor at the main hospital in Uganda, Dr. S, offered to take my blood samples and take them to the hospital for testing. He is the one who broke the news that I had sickle cell disease. This Dr was so helpful to Grandma because he would come with malarial injections from the hospital for me when I got malaria. We had support from the villagers because, before the diagnosis, everyone had ideas of what the illness could be. We lived in an extended family but when I got ill, everything would be at a standstill as it used to be so bad.

One would ask me why I am telling this story, but I want those who are in the same boat as my grandma was before I was diagnosed; to try and get medical attention, to be tested so that they know what you are dealing with. Furthermore, I would love those with children with sickle cell disease to know that the disease is not a curse; it's not a problem for the mother of the child/children with the disease, as we all know that it takes two to tangle. Sickle cell disease is an inherited disease. Both parents must have the gene to have a child with sickle cell disease. If one parent has the gene, there are chances that the child/children will have the trait. I would ask everyone to please go to hospitals for tests before having babies; baby screening is very important. Baby screening is the test done when babies are born. It's best to know earlier than to be in the dark.

I am writing about sickle cell because if at all, there is a young person with sickle cell who gets some complications but doesn't know about them, if they read this information, they can relate instead of being so worried.

Sickle cell patients should speak out so that health professionals and researchers can help to improve our lives by finding new ways of improving the quality of lives of many, maybe by finding new interventions that can prevent some complications.

Sickle cell disease is defined as a group of inherited haemoglobin disorders that are characterised by a high proportion of abnormal sickle haemoglobin in erythrocytes (Ndeezi et al 2016). In simple words, sickle cell disease is an inherited disease that affects the shape of the red blood cells, where they are half-shaped or like a banana or a crescent moon; since the sickle red cells are not full, they die off quicker than the normal cells in the body and this results into low levels of oxygen and become sticky in the veins, causing painful crises.

Sickle cell disease is a big health burden in the world, where almost 312000 babies are born with the disease every year. It is believed that 75% of this health burden of sickle cell is in sub-Saharan Africa (Tusuubira et al 2018).

The World Health Organisation explains that there is a great need for baby screening prevention and awareness of sickle cell disease (WHO, 2010).

According to National Institute for Health and Care Excellence (NICE), in 2016/17; 274 babies in England with sickle cell disease were detected by the National Health Service (NHS) screening for sickle cell disease and thalassaemia programme and 8530 babies with sickle cell trait. Furthermore, about 12,500–15,000 people have sickle cell disease in England alone (NICE 2021). While in Uganda, it is estimated that 20,000 babies are born with sickle cell disease every year but those are known ones and registered by the hospitals. There is no accurate data about the numbers (Ndeezi et al 2016) as some children are born through traditional birth attendants and do not get registered or screened.

Sickle cell disease is mostly common among African and African-Caribbean origin; however, it also happens in families from South and Central America; the Middle East, parts of India, and the eastern Mediterranean, and this may be because these places have a history of malaria migrated from the areas that are affected by Malaria.

Ethnic groups with a clinically significant prevalence of "haemoglobin S" include North Africans, African Caribbeans, Black British, African - Americans, those from Central and South America who have African ethnicity, and people from Italy, especially from Sicily, Greece, Turkey, Arabs, and India. Furthermore, due to intermarriages and migration, sickle cell disease is a clinical problem worldwide.

People living with sickle cell disease face more problems than just the effects the disease carries with it, for example, the stigma and being discriminated against (Tusuubira et al 2018) in the society that they live in. As a result, families with sickle cell patients tend to keep it a secret that they have family members with the disease (Tusuubira et al 2018).

The healthcare system in Uganda is totally different from that of England. In Uganda, to call for an ambulance, one must have money ready. Without money, an ambulance can't take the patient. To get treatment, you have to pay first, yet more than half the population cannot afford health care services. If a patient is admitted to a hospital, they must pay for the bed daily; one has to find food for the patient; medicine is for buying, and if the patient needs blood, the relatives of the patient have to go to the blood bank and find the blood.

Most sickle cell patients have sickle cell attacks and can't afford to go to hospitals as they don't have the funds. People resort to local herbs and buy a few tablets from pharmacies. This prolongs the time the attack takes to wear off and sometimes leads to death. While in the UK, I can call an ambulance at any time of the day.

I used to be admitted to hospitals every month while I was in Uganda. Sometimes I would be at school and the attacks started. I used to feel so sad as some of my peers would not understand what was wrong with me. Some would be bothered and worried, and some would even laugh; some would say that I got ill because I did not know how to pray and many more things. Sometimes I would be home and my attacks would be strong at night, but I thank God that my dad always took me to the hospital in whatever circumstances. No matter what time of the day or night, he would rush me to the hospital. I don't take that for granted and I am forever grateful. My dad never ignored my pain. I would sometimes see the stress in his eyes, but he always took me to the hospital without fail. In the UK, my husband took up that role. It does not matter the time of day or night; my husband makes sure that I have reached the hospital, and although he stays home without "triplets", he makes sure that I am safe and being looked after well in the hospital. Throughout my entire life, I have never sat down to think of the way my carers are affected by illness. Guess what? they get affected psychologically as they cannot take away my pain. My carers are warriors in their own respect. I treasure them so much as it's not easy to see your loved one screaming in pain. Special thank you to my grandma (RIP), my daddy (RIP) and my dear husband. They have been my main carers since the journey with my sickle cell anaemia began. I will never stop praising my grandma as she led the race in life. She took me when I was nine months old, fed me, dressed me, and put up with my illness until I was sixteen when my daddy took over the responsibility. My husband has stood by me on this journey without hesitation. As an English man, he did not know about sickle cell disease because it is not very common among Caucasian communities. I told him about it immediately after we met each other, as I did not want to waste his time and I did not want to be heartbroken, but I was surprised when he told me that it was ok; he was ready for it. Deep down, I thought he was playing games with me, and I did not have to wait long until I had a sickle cell attack. I was so terrified that he was going to leave me because that was a massive attack where I was just screaming in pain. He called an ambulance for me, and we went to the hospital. And he did not leave me alone. He even wanted to learn more about the disease and sixteen years later, we are still together, and he is my rock. I can never take this lightly as many would maybe feel overwhelmed and leave me. The friends I have met in the UK are so kind to me, and those that know about my illness, are so understanding and supportive. I have made the UK my home and would love it to be my resting place when I put down the button.

Hospitals in Uganda used to do their best but with the fewer resources in the health sector, the doctors never thought of examining the painful hip joint that I had since I was seven years old. I always complained of chest pain, but my doctors had never thought of or even heard of acute chest syndrome. According to Field &Willen (2022), acute chest syndrome is a severe lung complication caused by sickle cell disease and affects both children and adults with the disease.

Acute chest syndrome is like pneumonia, where the blood vessels in the lungs are blocked by the sickled red cells, which makes breathing so painful (Klings & Steinberg 2021). Acute chest syndrome is life-threatening and one of the leading causes of death in sickle cell patients. Chest infections exacerbate acute chest syndrome, and it leads to shortness of breath, low levels of oxygen, etc. When I came to England, that's when I understood the extent to which sickle cell disease had affected my body. I had a hip replacement; I got diagnosed with acute chest syndrome; my hip was replaced with a metal as the bone was wasted away by sickle cell disease; I was diagnosed with retinopathy, and so on.

Retinopathy is when the blood vessels in the retina become blocked, leading to the retina's thinning and abnormal blood vessel growth behind the eyes. Of course, there are gaps in the health care system in the UK regarding the knowledge of the disease and how best it can be treated. This may be because of the novelty of the disease in Europe. Research is not enough and the existing one is not updated since sickle cell affects every patient differently, and some health workers do not understand it as it is not entirely taught at universities. Since migration and intermarriage are happening, more attention is needed to train health professionals about sickle cell disease and sickle cell trait.

We are lucky that we have the National Health Services in England, which is a treasure to many, including me. Medical help is there if I need it. I have so many complications because of sickle cell disease but I always get the help I need. Of course, improvements need to be made, but it is much better than what I experienced when I was growing up in Uganda. In Uganda, when I would get admitted into a hospital, the medicine needed would have to be bought in a pharmacy far away from the hospital, the blood bank is so far away from the hospital and there is never blood and sometimes, the bribe has to be paid to those working in the blood bank, to get the blood. I was twelve years old, living in Uganda, when I had my first blood transfusion. I do not remember much about it, as I was mostly unconscious. That sickle cell crisis is one of the biggest crises that I have experienced.

In Uganda, if a family with a person with sickle cell disease has no car, then it's harder to reach hospitals and not everyone can afford the money for an ambulance. People struggle to take their loved ones to hospitals and when they reach there, help is mostly at hand if they have money. The problem of corruption plays a big part in this. To be attended to quickly, one must pay *kidongo kidogo (money in the form of a bribe)*. Blood is supposed to be free, but to get it as quickly as needed, you must pay those who work at the blood bank, which is not the case in England. When the doctors notice that I need a blood transfusion, they just talk to me and I sign the paperwork, and blood would be hooked on me at the time they said it would. I am so thankful to the doctors, nurses and all those who are involved in caring for me. One might say that it's their duty, but I can assure you that my health professional go beyond their duty to keep me alive and safe for as long as they can. I will never be able to thank them all, but I am forever grateful.

While I was in Uganda, hydroxyurea was not yet available there and there were no solutions apart from pain relief and drips. Today, hydroxyurea is available but costly, meaning those who cannot afford it are being left out. Blood exchange therapy is not common there yet; I imagine it would be very expensive. When I came to England,

I was introduced to hydroxyurea towards the end of 2005. When I came to England, my HB levels were so low. I would get a one-off blood exchange when I was impatient. This used to help me a lot. It would help me feel better and get a bit of energy. It would literally pick me up from the mouth of a grave. Hydroxyurea did not agree with my body. It made me feel weaker; I used to have bleeding gums, I used to have constant nausea, my quality of life was zero, I used to have bad breath, and my urine smelt like a medicine factory. In that process, I met my husband, William, and we fell pregnant so soon. I remember when I was a little girl in Uganda; I was always told that people with sickle cell disease do not get children. I did not realise I was pregnant and continued taking my hydroxyurea as normal. When I realised, I was pregnant, I was rushed to the hospital because I did not know what damage the medicine had done to the unborn baby. Those days, research about that medicine had only been done on animals and their babies were deformed due to that medicine. The medicine was immediately stopped, and talked about what could happen/could have happened already, and termination was discussed, which left me mortified. In my religion and my upbringing, termination is a sin. This stressed me so much, but I was worried about having a child with medical problems due to my health issues. I did not know what to do, but William held me up and took the lead in the matter. I, William, and the doctors had talks and agreed that the pregnancy could be monitored, and if the unborn baby develops any complications, we will terminate the pregnancy. I felt better and agreed to that, and my pregnancy was closely monitored; where I had a scan every two weeks until I got so ill that I had an emergency Caesarean at 36 weeks. I knew I was in good hands as I was allowed to have two birth partners. My husband and my friend/ sister KK.

My baby girl was perfect. She had all her fingers, toes, and face perfectly. I did not think I would make it out of the theatre and make a full recovery. I had a strong feeling that I was going to die.

I told my husband that our baby should be called Malayika, meaning Angel.

I don't remember the first two weeks of her life, as I was fighting a sickle cell crisis.

Hydroxyurea did not help me that much and had strong after-effects on my body, so I told the doctors to stop giving it to me. I was advised by the doctors to take a break from it to clear my mind. When I stopped taking medicine, I got ill very often. I talked to the doctors to try blood exchanges for me, as they had done it a few times for me as an inpatient. Unfortunately, blood exchanges were not yet researched and understood enough to be given often in the U.K. One day, I was called by the hospital to try regular blood exchanges. I was so happy to give it a go, and guess what? It was not a straight road either. Since my veins are thin and they collapse easily when in pain, it was a challenge for the health care workers to cannulate me. I would have central lines in my groins and neck but that also got to a point where the big veins got worn out. One day in 2013, I went for my Red Cell Exchange at the hospital; the central line was put in the groin for the procedure, it was removed safely, and I went home. About two hours later, I got up to go downstairs for my dinner, I started bleeding from the groin, and the vein had opened. This was a scary experience, but my husband was around, and he helped me to stop the bleeding and he called the ambulance. Due to fear and anxiety, I asked the doctors to stop the central lines for me. That's when I was given the choice of a double-lumen vortex port, which was a miracle for me. It is used for my Red Cell Exchange, drips, and medicine infusion.

I know that sickle cell disease will overpower my body one day, but I know I have fought a good fight and one day, I will rest from it all. However, I would like to raise as much awareness as possible to see the younger generation with this dreadful disease get better help when they go to the hospital for medical attention, and I would like them to have many medicinal options and a cure.

I would love to say a massive thank you to all the blood donors from all over the world for their kindness. They are helping us to have a bit of quality of life. A big thank you to all the health professionals under the sun. You are amazing, and to all the caregivers of people with sickle cell disease. It is not an easy day-to-day task but thank you. There are those relatives who have passed on and cannot say thank you anymore; I am saying it on their behalf.

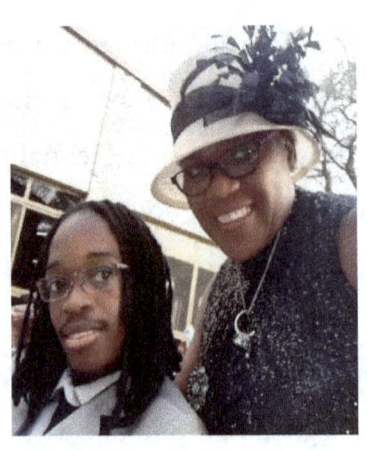

A Mother's Journey with Sickle Cell Disease and the Power of Community Support and the need for Mindset change
Sylvia Bwalya Mwansa-Caregiver

Introduction

Sylvia B Mwansa holds a Master of Business Administration International (MBA (I) from Edith Cowan University, Australia. Her Unique Value Proposition is that she is an Organizer, Effective and Efficient Communicator, who believes in bringing out positive attributes in self and others with a total belief that 'There is enough for everyone'.

Nicknamed "Sunshine" because of her happy character, Sylvia has been an entrepreneur for 3 decades. After she discovered that her son had sickle cell, she quit her formal job to start a business so that she could be able to use her time without restrictions and able to take care of Chileshe. Sylvia owes being an entrepreneur to Chileshe Stephen Mwansa, her Warrior! She is the Founder and CEO of SBM

(Simply Best Merchandise) Investment Limited est. 1994 which has enabled her to be a leader in the Fashion Industry with numerous plaudits including dressing Presidents, First Ladies and VIPs. Passionate about etiquette that teaches those who need it for public office and or for personal knowledge. Her business portfolio extends to printing and advertising solutions in addition to Consulting: Change Agent, Facilitator/Teacher, Executive and Leadership (Personal & Business) Life Coach with Neural Linguistic Practitioner (NLP).

Passionate about Women Empowerment with Leadership, Networking for Success, and being an active Change Agent, she has achieved many firsts: First Woman of Colour to lead as President of Ladies Circle International, 2004-Romania, 2005-Icelanda, 2006-The Netherlands, 2007-Estonia and made Life Member of Ladies Circle Zambia in appreciation. First Woman as Zambia Chambers of Commerce and Industry-Vice President in charge of Commerce & Trade up to 2021. A member of the Chartered Institute of Arbitrators (CIArB), A Fellow of the Institute of Directors (FIoD). A life-long learner and Teacher at heart, she has mentored many young men and women in business and in life skills. She was honoured by the United Nations Global Women Foundation with a Woman of Distinction Award.

Sunshine Sylvia is a completed doctoral candidate in Business Administration (DBA) at the Binary University, Malaysia in partnership with the University of Zambia. A wife, mother to a warrior (34-year-old) with four others and grandmother of 9 who is a firm believer in balancing her Wheel of Life in the six core areas of Family & Home, Physical & Health, Finance & Career, Social & Cultural Mental & Educational, as well as Spiritual & Ethical wellbeing which she facilitates to Leaders.

Sylvia is an Entrepreneur in Residence at the Lancaster University (LU), UK. In networking for success and love to serve those less privileged than herself in community service, Sylvia is a founder and President for Agora International in Zambia, a forerunner to Ladies Circle International. She is an international Distributor of the Jeunesse Global Wellness products that has changed her world in wellness, especially for Chileshe.

In the quest to see the change she expects and looks forward to, Sylvia has created a Change Management tool, "My Process to Mindset Change® Program' for Effective and Efficient Personal Time Management, Succession Planning, Retirement Preparedness and Customer Service together with the Process to Mindset Change Success Planner®. She has authored a book 'Mindset Change is Possible' with personal examples as a reference book. She is using this tool to share in the Sickle Cell community that a warrior and care giver can achieve anything that they need when the combined resources are put to good use at the right time and especially utilizing the time when the Warrior is feeling good out of a crisis. Her son suffered a stroke on the 18th of April 2023. She is using the proceeds of this book to raise funds to undertake a bone marrow transplant scheduled for India. She has been a passionate supporter of Sickle cell awareness for the last 34 years. Non-Executive Chairperson for the Zambian Network for Sickle Cell Amplified Voices and Advocacy (ZNSAVA) since 2021.

The Story of my son, Chileshe

34 years ago, 3 days before Xmas, Stephen and Sylvia had a bouncy baby boy, all smiles, and celebrations. However, 6 months down the line, their lives shifted to caring for a Sickle Cell Child. Sylvia's mother-in-Love when she tried to complain told her one straight question, "Why not you"? From that time, it's been Gratitude to the gift of God. Having a Sickle Cell Disease Warrior child has enabled Sylvia to connect to the world. Sylvia had to stop formal employment to be able to be flexible to look after our son. In the process, she became an Entrepreneur, Service in Charity work and Advocate for Sickle Cell Awareness in Zambia and Africa became a huge hobby. Through Mentorship and an author, facilitator, she has discovered that, a lot is possible in the Sickle cell space. Our family, both nuclear and extended family embraced the condition of our Chileshe and extended massive support to his day-to-day life that enabled him to live a very well and manageable life for the last 34 years. Chileshe is a graphics designer by profession and works at SBM Printing and Advertising Solutions as Head Designer. Chileshe had been well until the 18th of April, when he suffered a stroke. This stroke was taken on very quickly because of the voluntary work Sylvia does in the Sickle Cell space. She was able to connect to the Doctors, Blood bank and the laboratories for quick response. Without this connection, the story would have been very different. She may not even have been able to share this amazing story. Many warriors have lost their lives

because of the absence of required care in the adult hospital. This quick action has enabled Sylvia to be motivated to do more in helping to advocate, amplify the voices of those who may not be able to do so. Chileshe is Recovering well with weekly physio, diet, and strict supervision daily. However, Chileshe needs to undergo an overdue bone marrow transplant. We need in total $45,000 for the transplant, plus other costs e.g., the donor passage, parents, accommodation, and upkeep for not less than 3 months approx. $33,000 with estimated total costs of $78,000 to cover many things in India. As life can be, our lives have been in Service and Charitable work. In my over 35 years of Charity Work and Service (Ladies Circle International and Agora Club International and my Husband Dr Stephen Mwansa former Round Table, 41 Club and Rotarian, President of Chilanga), I/we have been 'Helpers' to others. This time around, (a very challenging undertaking) I have given myself to use my Talent of Facilitating Mindset Change Process® Program Workshops (Cocktail Chats with Sunshine Sylvia-Building Plan B for Retirement Preparedness and Succession Planning) and authored a book "Mindset Change is Possible" to raise funds for our son to receive Bone Marrow Transplant. Yes, an opportunity we have been looking for, has come to share our story to the world who will read this book. We are in the 'missing middle' however, I know it is possible!!

The moment my son was diagnosed with sickle cell disease at six months old was one of the most life-altering experiences for me as a mother. As I held my precious little boy in my arms, I didn't know what the future would hold, but I knew our lives would never be the same again. From that moment, our journey with sickle cell disease began. As a parent, it was a heartbreaking and terrifying realisation that my son would endure a lifetime of medical challenges and pain. One of the most challenging aspects of this journey has been managing my son's pain. He has experienced numerous episodes of acute pain, which can last for days and sometimes weeks. As a mother, it is unbearable to see my son in such agony, and I often feel powerless to help. When he was little, whenever he was in pain, sometimes I didn't know how to hold him as I feared that I would hurt him more. Seeing him in pain makes me struggle mentally, knowing I cannot do anything.

Another challenge has been dealing with the emotional and psychological impact of the disease. It is difficult for my son to see his peers involved in normal day-to-day activities, sports or outdoor activities while he has to sit on the sidelines or miss school due to illness. Sometimes, he feels isolated and alone, and as a mother, it breaks my heart knowing that he is going through such struggles, yet I cannot help him. He would like to play football with his peers but cannot afford to tire himself out because he would fall into a crisis; sometimes, he is too tired to walk around. However, despite all these challenges, my son continues to amaze me with his resilience and strength. He is a fighter, and his spirit and determination have helped him to overcome many obstacles that come with the disease.

Through this journey and his resilience, I have learned to advocate for my son and fight for him to receive the best medical care possible.

I have also found support from various organisations and individuals who understand the struggles we face daily. Through talking to these individuals, I learned a lot about the disease and found that some of the complications that my son has, others don't have and vice versa. I have also gained a greater appreciation for life, and I make sure to cherish every moment that I have with my family. As a mother, I am constantly reassured that I am doing my utmost to ensure my son lives the best life possible.

As a mother and caregiver to my son, who has Sickle Cell Disease, I have experienced first-hand the critical role that community support plays in the individual's and family's ability to cope with the challenges of SCD. As I mentioned when he suffered a stroke. One encouraging factor is that communities are beginning to embrace and understand the disease better, but there is still a long way to go.

When my son was first diagnosed, we felt alone and overwhelmed as very few people in our community knew about the disease, including ourselves as it was the first time, we were hearing about sickle cell disease, let alone how to support us. He used to ask me many questions as to why he is the only one among our children to suffer from SCD. After many years of supporting SCD as individuals, we discovered that there was much we could do and may get mileage in joining groups. It is for this reason that we discovered the Zambian Network for Sickle Cell Disease Amplified Voices and Advocacy, and I became its Non-Executive Chairperson. It was a turning point for us and many others in Zambia. It provided an opportunity for us to get our son to get tested to undergo a bone marrow transplant. The network provides free counselling services, support, and information for families affected by the disease. They also work to raise awareness of SCD in the community by holding sensitisation campaigns that target the general public, health professionals, and policymakers. In the long run, this will help so many families being affected by sickle cell disease by empowering them with support and information. Being a part of this community has given us a sense of hope and comfort, as we have been able to connect with people who understand our struggles and offer us practical advice on how to best manage the disease. Community support has also helped us to have a better quality of life as it has allowed us to lead a more fulfilling life. I believe that every patient with SCD and their families should have access to this kind of support. The more people in our communities who understand SCD, the more support we can provide to those living with the disease. This will mean that people with SCD can lead a more quality of life and have their full potential realised. The world needs to be more sensitised about sickle cell disease so sickle cell patients and their families can be better supported. This can be done by having more community organisations like the Zambian Network for Sickle Cell Disease Amplified Voices and Advocacy working together for a better SCD community.

To end my journey with my son's sickle cell disease has been challenging, but it has also been a learning experience. It is this experience that we offer to those being told after us that their children have sickle cell disease. The lessons we share are:

- Listen to the warrior.

- Know what works for them.
- Obey instructions from the clinicians.
- Keep warm when it's cold.
- Be in a well-ventilated space when hot.
- Take the correct doses of medication.
- Dehydrate often by drinking clean water. • Checkup as required for blood levels (HB) • Avoid infections.
- Prepare and feed on nutritious balanced meals.
- When a warrior agrees to go to the hospital, it's an emergency because you have done all the routine for pain treatment at home.

Being a care giver, has taught me to be a fierce advocate for my child and others, to appreciate life more, and to cherish the precious moments spent with my family. Above all, it has taught me to appreciate the resilience and strength that lie within us all. I thank my family for being there for our son. Whenever he is in hospital, everyone brings themselves to be useful by being empathetic and not sympathetic because sympathy does not solve anything. However, when you have empathy, there are solutions and care that one can bring to the table. Community support and empathy are essential for people with sickle cell disease and their families. Through community organisations such as the Zambian Network for Sickle Cell Disease Amplified Voices and Advocacy, families and patients can access much-needed information, counselling, and support. It is our hope as a family that more organisations and communities will prioritise understanding and support for those living with SCD. However, for us to manage the whole affair of Sickle Cell Disease, we need a Mindset Change. This is a process that can be developed starting now. How this can be done is shared after Chapter Six.

How can we shift Mindset in the Sickle Cell Space?

Mindset change refers to the process of deliberately shifting one's beliefs, attitudes, and perspectives towards a particular topic or situation. It involves recognizing and challenging existing thought patterns, assumptions, and limiting beliefs to adopt a new mindset that is more positive, empowering, and conducive to personal growth and development to tackle the sickle cell pandemic.

We are aware that mindset is a set of beliefs, attitudes, and assumptions that shape one's thoughts, behaviours, and reactions to various situations. It is the lens through which an individual views the world and themselves. A mindset change, therefore, involves consciously modifying this lens to adopt a new perspective.

Mindset change is not about simply changing one's thoughts in the moment, but rather about creating lasting shifts in one's beliefs and attitudes. It involves a deep and intentional examination of one's existing mindset, challenging its validity and usefulness, and actively working towards adopting a new and more supportive mindset.

Mindset change can have a significant impact on various aspects of life, including personal relationships, career goals, health and wellness, and overall well-being. By adopting a more positive and growth-oriented mindset, individuals can overcome obstacles, embrace challenges, and tap into their full potential. This will come by putting activities that change from what it is to what can be.

It is important to note that mindset change is not an overnight process and requires consistent effort, self-reflection, and practice. However, it can lead to long-lasting transformation and positive outcomes in six areas of life including change in family and home, financial and career, mental and educational, physical and health, spiritual and ethical and finally, Social and Cultural.

The mindset change process typically involves several key elements:

- Awareness: Acknowledging and becoming aware of the current mindset and its impact on thoughts, behaviours, and outcomes.
- Reflection: Reflecting on the beliefs and assumptions that underlie the existing mindset and considering their validity and usefulness.
- Challenge: Questioning and challenging existing limiting beliefs, self-doubt, negative thought patterns, and behavioural patterns.
- Re-framing: Identifying alternative perspectives and viewpoints that can lead to a more positive and empowering mindset.
- Learning and growth: Engaging in learning activities, seeking new knowledge and information, and adopting new strategies and behaviours that support the desired mindset change.
- Support and accountability: Seeking support from others, such as mentors, coaches, or support groups, and holding oneself accountable to the commitment of mindset change.

The mindset change process can be applied to various aspects of life, including personal relationships, career goals, health, and wellness, and coping with challenges or setbacks. It is based on the belief that by changing our mindset, we can improve our attitudes, beliefs, and behaviors, ultimately leading to improved outcomes and a more fulfilling life.

Conclusion

The mindset change process can play a significant role in improving the awareness and life of individuals affected by Sickle Cell Disease (SCD) in several ways:

1. Education and knowledge: The mindset change process can help increase awareness about SCD through education and knowledge dissemination. By providing information about the disease, its symptoms, treatment options, and management techniques, individuals affected by SCD can better understand their condition and make informed decisions.

2. Breaking stereotypes and reducing stigma: SCD is often accompanied by misconceptions and stigma due to a lack of awareness. A mindset change process can challenge these stereotypes and reduce the social stigma associated with the disease. By promoting acceptance, understanding, and empathy, individuals with SCD can feel more supported and less isolated.

3. Empowering individuals: The mindset change process can empower individuals affected by SCD by promoting a positive mindset and improving self-esteem. By focusing on the strengths and capabilities of individuals, rather than solely on the challenges they face, they can develop a sense of empowerment and agency in managing their condition.

4. Encouraging proactive self-care: The mindset change process can help individuals with SCD shift from a passive attitude to a proactive

approach towards managing their health. By emphasizing the importance of self-care practices such as sticking to treatment plans, maintaining a healthy lifestyle, and seeking appropriate medical advice, individuals can improve their overall well-being and reduce the frequency of disease-related complications.

1. Fostering resilience and coping mechanisms: Living with a chronic illness like SCD often requires individuals to develop resilience and effective coping mechanisms. A mindset change process can help individuals build resilience by promoting a growth mindset, encouraging positive thinking, and providing tools for managing stress, anxiety, and pain associated with the disease.
2. Promoting advocacy and support networks: The mindset change process can help individuals affected by SCD become advocates for themselves and others with the condition. By fostering a sense of community, individuals can engage in raising awareness, advocating for improved healthcare services, and connecting with support networks. This can create a support system that offers valuable emotional support, sharing of experiences, and access to resources.

Ultimately, by promoting a mindset change and empowering individuals affected by Sickle Cell Disease, the overall awareness and life quality of those with the condition can be improved.

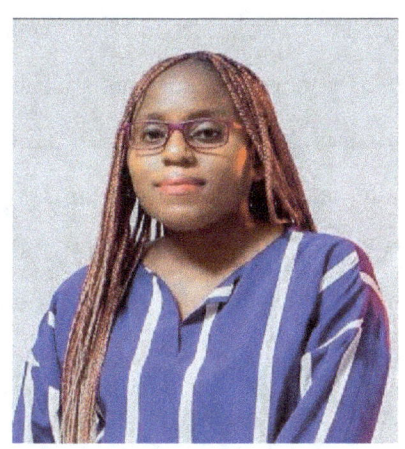

Sickle Cell Journey: From Struggles to Empowerment
By Verah Nambaya

My name is Verah Nambaya, I am a nurse by profession currently residing in Chingola, Zambia. I am a mother of four beautiful children, two boys and two girls. My third-born daughter, Jemimah happens to be a warrior. She is an intelligent, self-driven girl who wants to be a doctor when she grows up.

I am the fourth born in a family of six and I grew up in Ndola where I did both my primary and secondary school education. Growing up, I don't recall being nursed or admitted for any serious illness neither were my brothers or sister. I would say that I was a healthy child without any chronic illness.

I did learn the basics of genetics and Sickle Cell Disease in Biology, but my first real interaction with a person living with the disease was when I was a student nurse in 2007. One of our seniors had sickle Cell disease (SCD) and being in a school set up we were all affected in one way or the other. This was a person who would be fine at one time and then suddenly, you would see her friends panicking and taking her to the hospital while she screamed in pain. This had been her way of life especially before and during exams. I got so attached to her because she was such a determined person and never let Sickle Cell disease get in her way. Most of the time, she wrote her exams from the hospital bed but that didn't stop her, and she would pass. She was soft-spoken and one of the strongest people I have ever come across. She managed to complete her nurse's training, went on to do a degree and became a lecturer at one the biggest nursing colleges in Zambia. Unfortunately, she succumbed to sickle cell two years ago MHSRIP.

Having learnt about the disease and just seeing one of our friends suffering; my friends and I were prompted to go and have ourselves screened, unfortunately, at that time, electrophoresis one of the confirmatory tests was not being done. Out of curiosity, we only checked our blood groups and hemoglobin (HB) levels.

Time went by and I got married to the love of my life and had my own children. My first and second children are okay but my third and special child Jemimah was born in 2017. It was a normal delivery, and her weight was okay; generally, everything was okay. When she was five (5) months old, I noticed that she lost appetite, was irritable and could easily catch infections such as the common cold. She lost weight and I thought it was teething or reinfection from my other two children who were both under five years old and were in nursery. Every time she had a cough, it could not clear on its own not until I administered anti-biotic but even after completing the course, she would still get sick.

One morning, she woke up very irritable and looked quite weak. She had been coughing for almost two weeks and had poor appetite. I tried to breastfeed her, but she kept crying, and suddenly she "lost consciousness" for a few seconds or more. I quickly rushed her to the hospital where I worked. On our way, she seemed better, but we still decided it was best to go to the hospital.

At the hospital, she was examined by the medical doctor we were told that nothing was wrong with her. He jokingly said that maybe I had slept on her. I tried to explain to him what happened, but I guess it didn't just make sense. Anyway, I insisted that she be admitted so that she could be seen by the paediatrician and that was how she was admitted. I also requested that they check her full blood count (FBC). While we were in the ward, the paediatrician came through, and examined her but did not find any abnormalities. He advised me to give her small but frequent meals since I had mentioned that she had lost appetite and weight. He reassured me and discharged me on one condition that I should wait for the results. The results took longer than I had expected, and I became impatient because I had no one to look after my two older children who were at home. Finally, the results (FBC) were brought to the ward and being a member of staff, I grabbed them, when I closely looked at them, I could see that her HB was 6.4, and the white cell count was high. I had seen these kinds of results before and the first thing that came into my mind was Sickle Cell disease. I had worked in that ward. I started crying uncontrollably; in my mind, I knew my life was never going to be the same again. I had nursed children with Sickle Cell disease, and I knew how these children suffered, together with their parents or guardians. How some of them had died right before my eyes, the frequent admissions, the pain and probably the discrimination associated with the disease. I knew about one child who had become blind, lame, and dumb after suffering from a stroke. I remembered how I used to encourage their parents or guardians to put everything in God's hands each time their children were admitted. One mother came to my mind; she has 3 children and all of them are warriors. These children were in and out of hospital and at times, all of them would be admitted at the same time. When I was pregnant, she encouraged me to have more children because I was still young and had no genetic traits. That day was the longest day of my life, the entire staff on duty came to comfort me.

The paediatrician was called, and he came as quickly as possible, he had to re-examine my child and realized that she was pale and had a tinge of jaundice. He had put her on observation for another twenty-four (24) hours. He plainly told me that she had clinical features of sickle cell disease, but we needed to do a confirmatory test. Our hospital does not run this test, so it was outsourced to another laboratory in a different town. This meant that I had to wait for at least two more weeks for the result to be ready.

On the other hand, she was put on folic acid and Pen V. I had to call my parents to ask if at all they knew we had a trait from either my mother's side or my father's side, both had no idea. We asked my husband's family too, but we couldn't find any. Nevertheless, we just concluded to say that probably most of us were just carriers and it just happened that I got married to another carrier. I had so much going on in my mind. The following day we were discharged from the hospital. The days that followed being discharged, were like a nightmare to me. I became so depressed, and I lost a lot of weight within a few days. My husband's family denied that there was no way he could have a child with Sickle Cell disease because they had never heard of anyone with the disease from their side. However, I realized that my in-laws were ignorant about the condition hence I needed to help them understand that Sickle Cell disease is a genetic disorder, and it takes two carriers to produce a child with sickle cell disease.

I promised myself that I was going to research more about the disease, and I was going to do everything possible to improve my daughter's health and my marriage at large.

A few weeks later, the results came out and indeed Jemimah had Sickle Cell disease. Because I was eager to learn, the Doctor told me that there was a new drug on the market called hydroxyurea, and he advised me to read about it. I did read about it I thought that it was okay for my child to be commenced on it. I shared the idea with my loving husband who also agreed to it.

At exactly one year old, Jemimah was commenced on hydroxyurea. She responded so well that she has been on it since then and has only been admitted once to the hospital for a chest infection but has never been transfused for the past 5 years.

The greatest challenge that I am facing as a care giver is the non-availability of hydroxyurea. Many times, when the hospital fails to buy this drug, we have to buy them by ourselves which is very expensive. I have also noticed that people still don't have enough knowledge about the disease, and we have a lot of new cases within our community and at the hospital where I work. However, I came across a certain mother who is very passionate about SCD. She has two warriors, and she is a founder of a Sickle Cell club called Haven of Salem. Together with our hospital management, we started going round sensitizing people about the disease.

I came across the Zambia Sickle Cell group through Facebook, and I must confess, I have learnt a lot through this organisation. Keep up the good work.

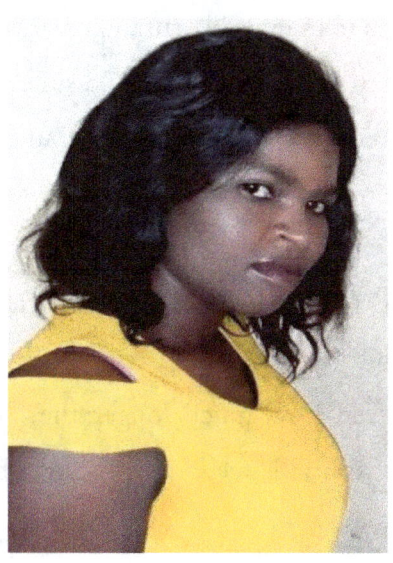

The Sickler Cell Warrior
By Wegginess Mwandila

The year was 1997, and we were living in Isoka, Muchinga Province of Zambia. I was only 3 years old then. My parents tell me this part of my story as I don't really remember any of it.

Apparently, I had an unexplainable, persistent stomach-ache. When the doctors eventually came back with a diagnosis, they said, "Your daughter has sickle cell anemia, the most severe form of sickle cell disease."

My parents were devastated. My mum cried the whole day and night after the diagnosis. Originally from Liberia, West Africa, they had only heard and seen nightmare tales of the sufferings and sudden deaths of people with Sickle Cell Anemia (SCA).

Diagnosed at age 3, before I knew what life was or why I had come to be, I was somehow keenly aware that I was not like everyone else around me. It was as if an invisible curtain encircled me. I could always tell by the way the grown-ups would sidle up to one another at family get-togethers and whisper, gesturing in my direction.

On good days, when I wasn't in much pain, I would bounce on my daddy's knee while we made funny faces and blew raspberries at each other. On bad days, I woke writhing in pain, often in the middle of the night, unable to stand and walk. I remember feeling betrayed by my body. I wondered how much longer the pain would last. In general, I had an inexplicable feeling that I didn't have as much time as those around me.

As my doctor appointments became more frequent, I became more and more curious about exactly how I was different from my family. I wanted to know why it seemed that as I grew older, I got fewer beaming smiles and more pursed lips of pity. I had always had a thirst for knowledge and as I grew into adolescence. By the time I got to high school, thanks to the dawn of the internet age, I discovered the grim reality of my situation.

It was September 7th, 2000, and I was admitted to the hospital then. I was admitted on August 8th, 2000. Eventually, I had to spend my birthday in the hospital. I was so sad, but my mom kind of threw me a birthday party! I was so excited because I didn't know what she was up to. She even had my friend planning it as well. She also has sickle cell ss type and was admitted to the hospital, and we were like 3 doors down from each other. It was the first time we had both gotten admitted at almost the same time. Me and my mom took her some cake and visited her for a bit. She even visited me and brought me chips and candy. I love her. She eventually got discharged, but she wasn't getting better and had to go to the infusion for pain management. She gave me a call and asked me if I wanted anything from the cafeteria and I got her to get me a few snacks from the vending machine. She was so sweet she had brought them after her visit and stayed for a good 30-40 minutes and we talked.

After that, I was really hoping to get out of the hospital sooner but I'm still fighting, and I'll never stop. But I just want to send a message to all my warriors and let you guys know that we are fighters and just because we can't always do certain things doesn't mean we can't become a nurse or lawyer whatever you want to just be yourself and thrive!! Remember we all got this and don't give up!

What little information I could find on sickle cell back then was immediately banked in my mental vault. With every new fact or noteworthy mention, I filled up on the knowledge of what was happening in my body. However, no matter the route, I still found myself arriving back at the same conclusion: my life would be a short one. And sadly, this explained the looks on all those faces.

I grew up during a time when a problem inside the family stayed within the family. My family knew I was born with a chronic disease, but I was simply a sick child to the community due to pride and privacy. I was not allowed to participate in activities that children in our neighbourhood enjoyed. For example, the fire department would open the fire hydrant for people to cool off during hot summer days, and everyone from young to old would enjoy getting wet while I watched on the steps of our building. I missed many school days, and when I was able to go to school, I was often set aside during recess and dressed in layers to stay warm out of worry that I could get a pain crisis.

When I was 11 years old, my mom, oldest sister, her wife, and I all moved to Nakonde, Muchinga Province of Zambia. When I tell you I had the worst pain I ever had in my entire life that I had to get admitted for at least a week and a half. I think it was due to us moving and the elevation was changing cause when I tell you I was in extremely so much pain, it was so excruciating. Eventually, I got better and finally could go home.

My grandmother and my faith have strongly influenced how I deal with Sickle Cell Anemia. My culture relies heavily on nature. I endured pain for many years and when I was young, the only medication I knew of was penicillin and folic acid. Growing up, my grandmother made vegetable juices; homemade syrups made with onion, radish, and honey; and plenty of pain salve to help manage my pain. These continue to be part of my regimen today. Other home remedies, such as rubbing over-the-counter ointments on my nose and the sole of my foot before going to bed and other ointments, were used to manage my pain. I have recipes to help me manage different complications or symptoms. Faith has always had a strong presence in my life.

Based on what they knew then, my life expectancy was set at 21 years, while my quality of life was expected to be interrupted by frequent hospitalizations, looking malnourished, and being ill all the time. The diagnosis truly took my parents by surprise because they never knew they were both carriers of the sickle cell trait until I showed up with the full-blown condition.

Sickle Cell Anemia is an inherited blood disease that causes red blood cells to be sickle- or crescent-shaped instead of round. These sickle-shaped blood cells do not live as long as healthy cells and can get stuck in blood vessels, leading to chronic anemia and oxygen shortage as the blood flow is obstructed. This obstruction is known as a vaso-occlusive crisis, or pain crisis, and can lead to severe joint pain, vital organ damage, and even death.

Growing up with sickle cell was so hard because you'd be sick so much and miss out on so many things like sports, spending time with friends, and going to parties you name it. Even though I couldn't do much like other teenagers I still had a great life. I still had opportunities; I danced for two majorette dance teams, attended after-school programs, and even did a bit of sorority with my god sister as well. I also did a little cheerleading and track in school but due to my sickle cell and asthma, I had to stop doing track and eventually had to stop cheering as well.

My mom always prayed with me, and she understood my pain. She made sure none of the nurses or doctors mistreated her baby girl, I always loved that because she showed me, she cared. She was there every time I would get admitted or even if I was in the emergency room.

Looking back on my childhood in Isoka, Muchinga Province of Zambia with Sickle Cell Anemia, all I remember are the rules I had to stick to, to avoid being hospitalized, and being raised to teach others around me about the illness to foster awareness, acceptance, and critical support when needed.

When I was 12 years old, Vanessa (my cousin) and I went to the Camp in Muyombe. It's a special memory because it was the first time we felt like normal kids. I was allowed to do things that my parents would not let me, like swimming, because they were worried it could lead to a pain crisis. At camp, we had an activity called "polar bear swimming," where we went into the pool in the morning and were given many heavy blankets when we got out of the pool to stay warm to help avoid a pain crisis. We also got to go camping and do woodworking. We met other kids with illnesses, not just kids with sickle cell Anemia. When everything seemed like a "no" for us, camp was where things were a "yes" with a medical team that could take care of us at any time. It was one of the best experiences growing up. After a few months in school, it was getting close to graduation and I kind of knew I wasn't going to graduate due to missing so much school from having so many pain crises. So, I found out that I didn't graduate, and I had to repeat the twelfth grade, but that was fine with me. I had to sign up for adult school which I finished up then and graduated.

So, about a year later, I started doing better, I was a junior in high school. I was doing so well that I had friends, good grades, I was even attending theatre for a few days. I had a pain crisis and couldn't perform due to sickle cell pain crisis when I told you I was so upset because I really wanted to do the play but had to stay home and I eventually went to the emergency room, and I had gotten admitted for two whole weeks. When I say I missed so much school that I was barely there due to sickle cell acting up so much. But I made sure I did the work and had it turned in every week even if I was sick, I still made sure I did my homework and got it done.

Deprived of a lot of normal day-to-day childhood activities, anything from field trips, team sports, friends, or family gatherings. I remember jazz recitals were coming up. They were on a Sunday, and I remember having a sickle cell crisis a couple of days beforehand. I had practiced so hard, and I was just absolutely devastated. I was so angry with myself. It wasn't even my fault, but I was so angry I could not attend that recital.

"The inability to do my normal day-to-day tasks still bothers me until this day. As soon as I know there's a sickle cell crisis coming on, I get so upset and so angry with it. I don't know. I just get so upset with my body and like, why now? Why are you doing this?

"So, I guess growing up, you know you can't do this, you can't do that, you'll never be able to do this or be able to do that. I guess I've become defiant towards my own disease in a sense. So, anything anybody tells me I can't do, I go out to try to do [it] anyways. I guess there's a part of me that is rebellious against my own disease and [wants to] see exactly how far I can go."

The turning point in my life was losing Vanessa. She was the only one I knew who shared my experiences. We were cousins, but, in my heart, we were sisters. She died at the age of 20 from pneumonia, a complication from her Sickle Cell Anemia. The experience of losing her was painful, but it taught me two lessons: (1) life is a precious gift, and (2) life is also a chance to live each day as if it is your last. After Vanessa's death, I fell into a deep depression, and my health declined. I experienced many pain crises. I was hospitalized frequently and needed many blood transfusions.

Since then, it has been hard living with sickle cell. From sickle cell crisis to depression and suicidal thoughts to a new way of life. Living with sickle cell has changed my life. It's made me see things most people don't. It makes me feel special like God loves me because I am different, and I know He will always be there for me.

I remember despising learning so much about this illness I never chose to have — one that I thought would in the best case, dominate my life, and in the worst case, terminate it.

The clothes I wore, the food I ate, and how much I drank all had to be seriously considered and planned daily, to avoid triggering a pain crisis or acute anemia — also known as aplastic anemia — because of low iron counts, dehydration, or exposure to extreme temperatures.

From a young age, I was faced with my own mortality. That may just be what shaped me to be a serious child.

Having sickle cell was so hard because I missed a lot of school, couldn't do certain activities, and had to take so many medications. I am part of a family of five and I'm the baby with two brothers and two sisters. My mom had the trait, but she never really had to be admitted or go to the hospital for any pain related to sickle cell. I'm also the only one out of all my siblings who has sickle cell disease.

My illness really affected me as a child, and my teenage life was bad. But, as I got older, I had better control and a clearer understanding of my body and signs. I feel like I went through a lot of my early teen years crying. I didn't have it in me to be rebellious, so I reverted to tears — tears of frustration, tears of isolation, tears of pain.

I was hospitalized more often than my peers because of Sickle Cell Anemia. Yet, I wasn't able or allowed to participate in those status-affirming sleepovers or class trips because of the risk of me getting sick, or worse —wetting my bed because of my required high-water intake, was too great.

Thank God, life started improving for me once I overcame the bedwetting, found my tribe of friends, and surrendered to the fact that I wasn't going to follow fashion and have my midriff on display for multiple reasons. Being hospitalized wasn't as depressing anymore, because I had friends to visit me and to look forward to hanging out with when I was discharged.

I love my team...anyway, I practice the all-natural way before I take any pain meds because, for me, it's all in your head. I know my signs and my body very well and it talks to me. At the top of my list is having a strong spiritual foundation. I do meditation, yoga, hot baths, aromatherapy, praying, massage therapy, and breathing techniques. I do all this and if it gets too bad, I will take meds, keep myself well-hydrated, and rest.

Then came my A-level years and getting my driver's license. Those were some of the sweetest years of my life. They combined my love for learning, the freedom from serious responsibilities, and the pleasure of being permitted to drive my mum's car and stay out until late.

I felt alive. I felt normal. I felt like I finally belonged. And then, my family moved to Ndola, Copperbelt Province, Zambia.

I always hated being classed as disabled, even though when the acute phases of Sickle Cell Anemia hit, I was undoubtedly just that. But, when it was time for me to apply to Copperbelt University (Zambia), I ticked the disabled box in my application. Although I enjoyed learning, the physical demands of academic life were simply too much for my sickly body.

In this journey. I've seen and experienced my own share of rejection, stigma, mood swings, depression, and suicidal thoughts. I hold on to God's Word and have a network of believers of God that help me remain resilient to live. I decided to use my story to encourage others struggling with other issues of life.

It has been a rollercoaster of emotions and trauma since childhood. As I little girl, I never understood why things I didn't sign up for would come my way. I remember nights when I'd cry myself to sleep with so many questions. Whose fault, was it? Who was responsible for the pain I had to endure during cold nights? Who was to blame for the way my heart would beat fast just because I had seen thunder strike or the clouds becoming darker and darker? Not to talk of the bullying. I was bullied by both students and teachers. Yes, teachers who would still give me strokes of canes each time I had crises claiming I was faking it. Who fakes that kind of pain? I question I'd constantly ask but would have no answer to.

Sickle Cell Anemia has a lot of limitations it poses on people living with it.... I've not been able to really spread out my wings the way I would have wanted to if I was free of Sickle Cell Anemia. For example, traveling is a problem for me, because I end up getting stressed out and ending up in the hospital, inconveniencing my host. I can't walk long distances; I can't stand up for more than 15 minutes without my back hurting deeply. So, mobility is another problem. In Zambia, standing to wait for the bus is a nightmare, because they'll push me down…they usually don't have patience for me. I have been through it all but my faith in God will not allow me to give up.

I try as much as possible to listen to my body, hydrate and not stretch myself too much beyond what I should.

The idea of being in a new Province (Copperbelt Province), living a 4-hour drive away from my parents for the first time, and no one knowing what I had going on was enough incentive for me to bury my pride and disclose my illness.

Building a new life in Kitwe, Copperbelt (Zambia), meant developing a new support system around me, and they certainly showed me how it should be done.

The Isoka's (Muchinga Province of Zambia) Sickle Cell Anemia literacy was much higher than Copperbelt's, and in my time there, I had a routine of seeing a haematologist a couple of times per year. I had the emergency oncology ward on speed dial, and I could connect with a community centre if I needed.

From my student years to when I was a full-time employee, I felt in safe hands, until I left the Copperbelt Province, Zambia. I've only ever had one actual boyfriend, and I'm married to him now. As much as it might sound romantic, that wasn't really by choice. But in the same way, I was mindful of my mortality as a child, which curbed some of my free-spiritedness, as a teen and young adult, I also knew I couldn't just go out or be with anyone.

From the age of 17, I'd been thinking about when the best time to disclose my chronic illness to a potential partner would be. By 21, I decided that I would need to know if my potential partner carried the sickle cell trait by taking a blood test before we caught feelings for each other. I would want to walk away to ensure my unborn children wouldn't also be doomed to a life with Sickle Cell Anemia.

At 24, I briefly toyed with the idea of giving up on having biological children altogether, as I was anxious about being pregnant in my 20s and what it might do to my health and life expectancy.

When my now-husband walked into my life 6 months before I turned 26, he was a true godsend. I told him about my condition on our second date, so he had ample time to walk away. He is a doctor, so he knew what he was letting himself for. He gladly obliged to take a blood test to get checked before we got serious. Since we've been married, he has been my biggest advocate and protector to ensure I keep my body from crisis-inducing activities, temperatures, and places. He also gives the best deep-tissue massages when I do have a pain crisis.

He's the perfect partner for me and my fight against Sickle Cell Anemia.

Following a terrible period of back-to-back pain crises triggered by immense work stress in 2019, my husband and I left Copperbelt Province and returned to Isoka, Muchinga Province. Since then, I have had the honour of working for myself in a role I love, with hours I can manage around my health.

Through my business, The Blueprint Way, I work as a qualified counselor and life coach, delivering online counseling and coaching services to millennial women of color seeking to 'live their best lives.' I also consult on various mental health and racial trauma-related projects, and I'm creating multiple streams of income and generational wealth through businesses with my husband.

The only area I still need to fearlessly embrace my identity and life with Sickle Cell Anemia is being a mother. Since being back in Isoka, Muchinga Province, I'm trying to create at least as good a support network around me as in the Copperbelt Province, before we try and have children.

Although Isoka still doesn't seem much further in their general knowledge of treating people with Sickle Cell Anemia, hopefully, time is on my side, and I will get things sorted before we even start trying.

As soon as I turned 21-22, I had to stop going to the children's hospital and I started going to an adult hospital. When I tell you I was so anxious, nervous, and scared because I'm so used to being at a children's hospital. When I had my very first visit to the adult hospital it was very a nervous moment for me, but I overcame it eventually when I met some nurses who were caring, especially

Racheal, she was so sweet and I'd never forget her. I always wanted her to be my nurse every time I would get admitted. Haha, funny right?

Living my best life...until the clocks run out.

I no longer see my Sickle Cell Anemia diagnosis as a fun-robbing childhood memory or an inconvenient life interrupter. Instead, I've learned to see it as my in-built self-care gauge. If my self-care tank is empty or close to it, the acute parts of Sickle Cell Anemia rear their ugly and very painful heads.

If I keep my self-care tank as full as possible, the chronic parts of Sickle Cell Anemia require much of the same standard most of our bodies do — a healthy, balanced lifestyle. I've always been a little obsessed with having a great quality of life. I guess it makes sense considering I was told from a young age that my life expectancy and quality of life would be low.

It also makes sense then, that I've always been meticulous about how I spend my time, especially the older I get. That's why I gratefully celebrate every single birthday I have because aging is a privilege that few recognize.

Now at age 28, I share my story to inspire other sickle cell warriors to open up and share their struggles, and I hope my story can help increase education and awareness of Sickle Cell Anemia in the Zambian community. I've travelled to Lusaka, Chipata, Solwezi, Monze, Kabwe, Nakonde, Chingola and Kasama, and connected with other sickle cell warriors from those areas. I inspire others with Sickle Cell Anemia to live a full and happy life by sharing my accomplishments as I earned my Bachelor of Science degree and had a great career as an Assistant Manager at The Skill Development Zambia.

I feel honoured to be a part of the important changes happening within the realm of Sickle Cell Anemia. I am currently serving on two committees researching methods for improving care for people living with Sickle Cell Anemia. One of my proudest moments was when I was invited to the Future of Hope Foundations and Your Youth Matters in 2021. I had the opportunity to share my personal experience living with Sickle Cell Anemia, and how it can affect a person's physical, mental, and emotional well-being. As a result, a resolution was passed to provide more funding for the Sickle Cell Treatment Act.

We, people with sickle cell, are born with a silent strength. The ability to endure pain upon birth is the validation that we can accomplish and overcome the challenges we face. Don't allow the illness to block your dreams. I hope we can raise more awareness of sickle cell disease, and with greater awareness comes more advances in care. I do pray there will be a cure someday so we all can have long lives, careers, and the stigmas of sickle cell disease stop.

Don't feel like you are in competition with anyone. Live your life at the speed it allows you to. Your journey is yours and you will end up getting to the finish line. It may be at a different pace than others, but you will get there.

I am a witness that even with this disease, you can accomplish so much in life, and believe it or not, you can accomplish much more than what others say you can't. I am a college graduate with a bachelor's degree in science. That was a major accomplishment because doctors were not expecting me to live past the age of 17.

I have successfully been gainfully employed with major companies while suffering from this major disease. I have sickle cell disease, but sickle cell disease does not have me. I have experienced many different life-altering events while managing sickle cell disease, but I thank God that I do not look like what I have been through.

Having been freed from the binds of sickle cell disease in so many ways, I now found myself most eager to live more than ever. I rededicated myself to warriors everywhere and I haven't looked back since. I learnt the hard way that no one could love me better than myself. Though I still have some insecurities, I do everything possible to rise after a fall and stay strong.

So, this piece is for anyone who feels lost and depressed to know that you're loved. Stay strong and do what makes you smile. Stay positive and make memories. It isn't easy but I believe in you. You can do it. Go you!

Only God knows when the clock will run out on me, but until then, I'll be focusing on living my best life.

— full of love, joy, freedom, and no regrets. And I'll continue to support, guide, and educate others to do the same.

Author; Wegginess Mwandila from Zambia.

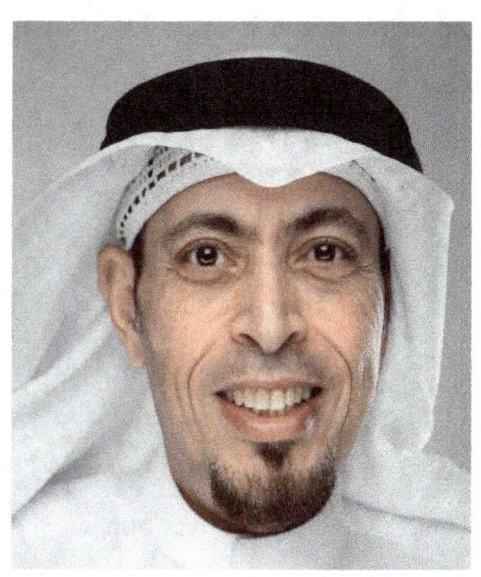

Sickle Cell Disease
By Zakareya Alkadhem

At the time of my birth, the doctors gave my mother a grim prognosis, saying that I would not live past the age of six. As I grew older, the predictions for my life expectancy continued to increase but never exceeded 42 years. However, today, at the age of 50, I stand before you, having defied the odds and surpassed all expectations. I have promised my children that I will continue to live a long and healthy life, with the hope of reaching the age of 75. Despite the uncertainties of life expectancy, I remain optimistic and grateful for every day that I am given.

Life and death and the association of death with sickle cell disease made me create my own philosophy.
My philosophy is the extension of the white lights that visited me 11 times in my life. These lights created amazement in my chest and

generated wisdom, from which I was able to extract meaning and help me reformulate my deep self.

When I was a child, I used to witness the pleasure in children's conversations and the adventure in their eyes. I was deprived of cycling, the sea, the pool, football, playing skating rinks, or I was deprived of wearing the clothes that suit me. I used to ask why. But I did not know that why is the most important question in every person's life and accompanies him throughout his life.

White lights visited for the first time when I was 18 years old, I can remember that night very well, I was lonely, weak, afraid, and confused. But I was very angry with my Lord, and I used to admonish him and say to him: "Am I the easiest of your servants to you because you give me a weak body and put in me a bad disease? Why?"

Today, as I stand before you, at the age of fifty, that scene is still present in my memory. I go back and ask myself: Really, I was the easiest of God's servants, when he put me in this disease? Between the age of 18 and today 50...the question is...Who am I today? Does anyone know my balance in the bank? Does anyone know my degrees? Relative? My post? No! But all Bahraini people and G.C.C know well that I live with sickle cell identity as patient No. 1 in Bahrain... everyone knows that I am the Godfather of 9,000 warriors, ... I carry their pains and aspirations and speak on their behalf in front of those concerned... I wear their uniform and represent their values and their morals.

How impressive it is to wake up in the morning and my phone is flooded with 16,000 messages from patients and mothers, to whom the doctors told them that their children will not live long... They see my life as an extension of their children's lives... They hope their children live as much as mine... As happy as I am... As successful as I am. What do they want from me every morning? All they want is for me to tell them that I am fine and that I will continue to live longer, happier and more successful. I discovered that 9000 people and their mothers' lives depend on me. Therefore, this made me slow in interpreting and explaining events, which gave me preference in choosing my emotions to be wiser and calmer... This allowed me to experience peace and tranquillity and earned me reverence, appreciation and reverence in the eyes of people.

Today, I am not allowed to err because I am the example, and I am not allowed to weaken because I am the hope.

I was born to a father who is a tradesman, and he is the best one who takes care of the pilgrims. He inherited it from my grandfather 80 years ago. He performed the duty as best as every father performs towards his children. It is time for him to rest and transfer this task to the children... And because I am the eldest, he said to me, I want you to complete the task and manage the affairs of the family. And it's trade. So, I apologized to him and said to him, Sir, I apologize to you, for I decided to live as a dervish as people are, a servant, not a master.

Go back and say why?

1. I can say that a person may die sad, even if he lived happily, because he did not meet the mission of his life and did not discover a reason for his upbringing.

2. And a person dies happy even if he lives miserably, but if he meets the mission for which God made him, even if it comes late.
3. But I was the happiest person when I met my mission early. God created us with a mission in the chest of every human being, and he must search for it. And throughout the journeys of life and death that I experienced 11 times in my life, and the talk of doctors and hopeless disease, I knew that I do not have the length of life, but I do have the capacity of life. They ask about the age of the deceased, how many great people do you know who lived 20, 30, or 40... but after 100 years have passed, 500 years, or a thousand or two thousand years, but his name is mentioned and well known throughout the world?

The truth is I am between living long or living immortal.
My grandmother, (Hilalah), may God prolong her life, says... My son, I don't want to die a cheap death... I asked her, what is a cheap death? She said that I would die on the bed of invalidity... I only want to die either standing by my family or serving my children.

This old lady gave me eloquent wisdom... and that is, if you want to die, die empty... die without idle responsibilities in your schedule... and if God wants to take me, then let him take me while I am in duty standing on the care of my children. And he will continue to build and protect the walls of the homeland and raise it.

The last visit to the White Lights was 5 years ago in the ICU room where 30 doctors surrounded me trying to bring me back to life.

And I could see the fear in their eyes and the lack of hope... So, I asked myself: Is this the last trip?

Is this the death they are talking about?

I am not afraid, worried, or angry, unlike the first time...
But it is the separation of loved ones.
The separation of loved ones
And meeting God is great... I will benefit from God, and I have nothing to present in God's hands as a greeting of presence... My account book is devoid of anything that can intercede for me... So, I conquered my Lord... My Lord, I bestow all the sins of Your servants to Your honourable face... May you accept me...and perhaps you will intercede for me with your servants in their rights over me.

While the doctors were busy bringing me back to life, behind them was a poor, strange Asian cleaner who was affected by what he saw and what he knew and did not know.

Within half an hour, the doctors' faces changed, and they congratulated this man, and they told me, "Thank God, you will live... Pray to God with gratitude."

By God, I do not know that my return to life was due to the skill of the doctors or the position of this poor, strange slave.

And then I asked myself... Did I need this ordeal to know the value of tolerance?
Did I need death to know the value of a person, no matter how poor or strange he is?
Sometimes, we think that we are the ones who have the credit for a person while he is the best for us.

Today, I have no Favor over my 9,000 children.
Rather, they are the ones who preferred me and accepted me as a courier servant... They were patient with my shortcomings and my extravagance.

They gave me their morals and knowledge, and they sat me down in their councils, so God raised me.

What I am going to say to you, my dear ones... I did not give specific answers... Rather, I awakened the question in your chest... And you will go back to your homes with the question moving in your chest... Many windows have opened.

Conclusion

Through these stories, we have all shown our emotions connected to SCD. These stories are from the sickle cell warriors, parents, and carers of the warriors, advocates, and healthcare professionals. Hopefully, this opens doors for many screening services, more research, and more training of the health professionals to listen to the patients and understand the warriors.

For policymakers, our hope is that these stories will help you to include favourable policies to reduce the burden of SCD, especially in issues like health insurance, prescription fees, and understanding warriors in workplaces without stigmatising them.

Sickle cell awareness is important to highlight the need to understand its effects on people's daily lives. When people with SCD read these stories, it brings a sense of belonging and comfort because they know, they are not alone in this journey. The unpredictable nature of the disease and the need to manage the symptoms is challenging for everyone, especially when it comes to attending school, working constantly, which affects the financial side, and being socially active is so hard, which brings on a part of loneliness.

Life is hard to balance with SCD because regular hospital visits are time-consuming and emotional challenges. For advocates, our hope is that you recognise the need for us to unite to fight this condition collectively. There is so much work needed to do to improve advocacy, services, education etc such that working together is the only key.

We would like to thank you for taking your time to read our stories. Should you have any questions, contact the book publisher, the details are on the first page. Should you wish to be included in volume three of such stories, contact the book publisher as well. Thank you and continue to live a healthy lifestyle.

REFERENCES

Field J.J & Willen S (2022) Acute chest syndrome (ACS) in sickle cell disease (adults and children)

Klings E.S & Steinberg M.H (2021) Acute chest syndrome of sickle cell disease: genetics, risk factors, prognosis, and management Expert Review of Hematology, DOI: 10.1080/17474086.2022.2041410

Ndeezi G, Kiyaga C, Hernandez AG, Munube D, Howard TA, Ssewanyana I, Nsungwa J, Kiguli S, Ndugwa CM, Ware RE, Jane R. Aceng (2016) burden of sickle cell trait and disease in the Uganda sickle surveillance study (US3): a cross-sectional study lancet global. Health. 4:e195–200.

NICE (2021) sickle cell disease: What is it?

Tusuubira, S.K., Nakayinga, R., Mwambi, B; Odda J; Kiconco, S & Komuhangi, A Knowledge, perception and practices towards sickle cell disease: a community survey among adults in Lubaga division, Kampala Uganda. *BMC Public Health* **18**, 561. https://doi.org/10.1186/s12889-018-5496-4

WHO (2010) Sickle-cell disease: a strategy for the WHO African region. Report AFR/RC60/8. Geneva: World Health Organization.

Adio, W.S., Christopher, F.C., Adesola, R.O. and Mary, F.I., 2022. Current trends in the treatment of sickle cell anemia. *World News of Natural Sciences*, *43*, pp.60-75.

Angastiniotis, M., Vives Corrons, J.L., Soteriades, E.S. and Eleftheriou, A., 2013. The impact of migrations on the health services for rare diseases in Europe: the example of haemoglobin disorders. *The Scientific World Journal, 2013*.

Ali, M.A., Ahmad, A., Chaudry, H., Aiman, W., Aamir, S., Anwar, M.Y. and Khan, A., 2020. Efficacy and safety of recently approved drugs for sickle cell disease: a review of clinical trials. *Experimental hematology*, *92*, pp.11-18.

Ballas, S.K., 2020. The evolving pharmacotherapeutic landscape for the treatment of sickle cell disease. *Mediterranean Journal of Hematology and Infectious Diseases*, *12*(1).

Biswal, S., Rizwan, H., Pal, S., Sabnam, S., Parida, P. and Pal, A., 2019. Oxidative stress, antioxidant capacity, biomolecule damage, and inflammation symptoms of sickle cell disease in children. *Hematology*, *24*(1), pp.1-9.

Brown, M., 2012. Managing the acutely ill adult with sickle cell disease. *British Journal of Nursing*, *21*(2), pp.90-96.

Crow, A., 2020. Transcranial Doppler in children with sickle cell disease: Five years of screening experience. *Australasian Journal of Ultrasound in Medicine*, *23*(1), pp.39-46.

Crighton, G., Wood, E., Scarborough, R., Ho, P.J. and Bowden, D., 2016. Haemoglobin disorders in Australia: where are we now and where will we be in the future? *Internal medicine journal*, *46*(7), pp.770-779.

Darbari, D.S., Sheehan, V.A. and Ballas, S.K., 2020. The vaso-occlusive pain crisis in sickle cell disease: definition, pathophysiology, and management. *European journal of haematology*, *105*(3), pp.237-246.

Ethier, I., Cho, Y., Hawley, C., Pascoe, E.M., Roberts, M.A., Semple, D., Nadeau-Fredette, A.C.,
Wong, G., Lim, W., Sypek, M.P. and Viecelli, A., 2020. P1431 MULTI-CENTER REGISTRY
ANALYSIS COMPARING SURVIVAL ON HOME HEMODIALYSIS AND KIDNEY
TRANSPLANT RECIPIENTS IN AUSTRALIA AND NEW ZEALAND. *Nephrology Dialysis
Transplantation*, *35*(Supplement_3), pp.gfaa144-P1431.

Ellis, J., Garner, E., Webster, K.E., Darzins, S., Galea, M.P. and Scheinberg, A., 2022. Establishing an Australian pediatric spinal cord disorder register using consumer, health professional, and researcher perspectives. *The Journal of Spinal Cord Medicine*, pp.1-9.

Farooq, S. and Testai, F.D., 2019. Neurologic complications of sickle cell disease. *Current neurology and neuroscience reports*, *19*, pp.1-8.

Feng, J.L., Hickling, S., Nedkoff, L., Knuiman, M., Semsarian, C., Ingles, J. and Briffa, T.G., 2015. Sudden cardiac death rates in an Australian population: a data linkage study. *Australian Health Review*, *39*(5), pp.561-567.

Galvin, J., Scheinberg, A. and New, P.W., 2013. A retrospective case series of pediatric spinal cord injury and disease in Victoria, Australia. *Spine*, *38*(14), pp.E878-E882.

Greenway, A.L., Kaplan, Z., Barbaro, P., Carter, T., Teo, J. and Pal, M., 2022. Benchmarking Paediatric Sickle Cell Care in Australia. *Blood*, *140*(Supplement 1), pp.5456-5457.

Henry, E.R., Metaferia, B., Li, Q., Harper, J., Best, R.B., Glass, K.E., Cellmer, T., Dunkelberger, E.B., Conrey, A., Thein, S.L. and Bunn, H.F., 2021. Treatment of sickle cell disease by increasing oxygen affinity of hemoglobin. *Blood*, *138*(13), pp.1172-1181.

Herity, L.B., Vaughan, D.M., Rodriguez, L.R. and Lowe, D.K., 2021. Voxelotor: a novel treatment for sickle cell disease. *Annals of Pharmacotherapy*, *55*(2), pp.240-245.

Hussein, N., Henneman, L., Kai, J. and Qureshi, N., 2021. Preconception risk assessment for thalassaemia, sickle cell disease, cystic fibrosis and Tay-Sachs disease. *Cochrane Database of Systematic Reviews*, (10).

Inusa, B.P., Hsu, L.L., Kohli, N., Patel, A., Ominu-Evbota, K., Anie, K.A. and Atoyebi, W., 2019. Sickle cell disease—genetics, pathophysiology, clinical presentation and treatment. *International journal of neonatal screening*, *5*(2), p.20.

Kanter, J., Liem, R. I., Bernaudin, F., Bolaños-Meade, J., Fitzhugh, C. D., Hankins, J. S., Murad, M. H., Panepinto, J. A., Rondelli, D., Shenoy, S., Wagner, J. E., Walters, M. C., Woolford, T. L., Meerpohl, J. J., & Tisdale, J. F. (2021). American Society of Hematology 2021 guidelines for sickle cell disease: stem cell transplantation. Blood

Advances, 5(18), 3668–3689. https://doi.org/10.1182/bloodadvances.2021004394c

Jonassaint, C.R., Shah, N., Jonassaint, J. and De Castro, L., 2015. Usability and feasibility of an mHealth intervention for monitoring and managing pain symptoms in sickle cell disease: The Sickle Cell Disease Mobile Application to Record Symptoms via Technology (SMART). *Hemoglobin*, *39*(3), pp.162-168.

Kahindo, C.K., Mukuku, O., Wembonyama, S.O. and Tsongo, Z.K., 2022. Prevalence and factors associated with acute kidney injury in sub-Saharan African adults: a review of the current literature. *International journal of nephrology*, 2022.

Kato, G.J., Piel, F.B., Reid, C.D., Gaston, M.H., Ohene-Frempong, K., Krishnamurti, L., Smith, W.R., Panepinto, J.A., Weatherall, D.J., Costa, F.F. and Vichinsky, E.P., 2018. Sickle cell disease. *Nature reviews Disease primers*, *4*(1), pp.1-22.

Kaur, M., Dangi, C.B.S. and Singh, M., 2013. An overview on sickle cell disease profile. *Asian J Pharm Clin Res*, *6*(1), pp.25-37.

Kazankov, K., Barrera, F., Møller, H.J., Rosso, C., Bugianesi, E., David, E., Ibrahim Kamal Jouness, R., Esmaili, S., Eslam, M., McLeod, D. and Bibby, B.M., 2016. The macrophage activation marker sCD 163 is associated with morphological disease stages in patients with non-alcoholic fatty liver disease. *Liver International*, *36*(10), pp.1549-1557.

Kumar, A.A., Chunda-Liyoka, C., Hennek, J.W., Mantina, H., Lee, S.R., Patton, M.R., Sambo, P., Sinyangwe, S., Kankasa, C., Chintu, C. and Brugnara, C., 2014. Evaluation of a density-based rapid diagnostic test for sickle cell disease in a clinical setting in Zambia. *PloS one*, *9*(12), p.e114540.

Lattanzi, A., Camarena, J., Lahiri, P., Segal, H., Srifa, W., Vakulskas, C.A., Frock, R.L., Kenrick, J., Lee, C., Talbott, N. and Skowronski, J., 2021. Development of β-globin gene correction in human hematopoietic stem cells as a potential durable treatment for sickle cell disease. *Science translational medicine*, *13*(598), p.eabf2444.

Lim, M.A.W.T., Liberali, S.A.C., Calache, H., Parashos, P. and Borromeo, G.L., 2021. Perceived barriers encountered by oral health professionals in the Australian public dental system providing dental treatment to individuals with special needs. *Special Care in Dentistry*, *41*(3), pp.381-390.

Liyoka, C.C.M., Suzanna, M., Birbeck, G., Nkole, L.K., Nanyangwe, A., Lupumpaula, C., Chilima, J.S., Kabemba, P. and O'Brien, N.F., 2022. Implementation of Transcranial Doppler Ultrasound Stroke Risk Screening in Urban and Rural Sickle Cell Disease Clinics in Zambia. *Blood*, *140*(Supplement 1), pp.7900-7901.

Makoni, M., 2021. Newborn screening for sickle cell disease in Africa. *The Lancet Haematology*, *8*(7), p.e476.

Manwani, D. and Frenette, P.S., 2013. Vaso-occlusion in sickle cell disease: pathophysiology and novel targeted therapies. *Blood, The Journal of the American Society of Hematology*, *122*(24), pp.3892-3898.

Muzazu, S.G., Chirwa, M., Khatanga-Chihana, S., Munyinda, M. and Simuyandi, M., 2022. Sickle Cell Disease in Early Infancy: A Case Report. *Pediatric Health, Medicine and Therapeutics*, pp.377-383.

Minniti, C.P., Knight-Madden, J., Tonda, M., Gray, S., Lehrer-Graiwer, J. and Biemond, B.J., 2021. The impact of voxelotor treatment on leg ulcers in patients with sickle cell disease. *American Journal of Hematology*, 96(4), p.E126.

Matte, A., Zorzi, F., Mazzi, F., Federti, E., Olivieri, O. and De Franceschi, L., 2019. New therapeutic options for the treatment of sickle cell disease. *Mediterranean journal of hematology and infectious diseases*, 11(1).

Matte, A., Cappellini, M.D., Iolascon, A., Enrica, F. and De Franceschi, L., 2020. Emerging drugs in randomized controlled trials for sickle cell disease: are we on the brink of a new era in research and treatment?. *Expert Opinion on Investigational Drugs*, 29(1), pp.23-31.

Molter, B.L. and Abrahamson, K., 2015. Self-efficacy, transition, and patient outcomes in the sickle cell disease population. *Pain Management Nursing*, 16(3), pp.418-424.

Musowoya, R.M., Kaonga, P., Bwanga, A., Chunda-Lyoka, C., Lavy, C. and Munthali, J., 2020. Predictors of musculoskeletal manifestations in paediatric patients presenting with sickle cell disease at a tertiary teaching hospital in Lusaka, Zambia. *Bone & Joint Open*, 1(6), pp.175-181.

Nwanonyiri, D.C., 2018. *Sickle Cell Disease in Children: An Exploration of Family Resilience through the Experiences of Family Caregivers* (Doctoral dissertation, Kean University).

Neumayr, L.D., Hoppe, C.C. and Brown, C., 2019. Sickle cell disease: current treatment and emerging therapies. *Am J Manag Care*, *25*(18 Suppl), pp.S335-43.

Oudin Doglioni, D., Chabasseur, V., Barbot, F., Galactéros, F. and Gay, M.C., 2021. Depression in adults with sickle cell disease: a systematic review of the methodological issues in assessing prevalence of depression. *BMC psychology*, *9*, pp.1-14.

Parise, L.V. and Berliner, N., 2016. Sickle cell disease: challenges and progress. *Blood, The Journal of the American Society of Hematology*, *127*(7), pp.789-789.

Salinas Cisneros, G. and Thein, S.L., 2020. Recent advances in the treatment of sickle cell disease. *Frontiers in physiology*, *11*, p.435.

Siachisa, M., 2020. *Administration of health services and challenges in the management of the prevention and control of malaria in Zambia: the case of Luangwa district* (Doctoral dissertation, The University of Zambia).

Simwangala, K., Tsarkov, A., Petlovanyi, P. and Paul, R., 2022. Exploring neurocognitive deficits among children with sickle cell disease and its impact on their quality of life at the University Teaching Hospital, Lusaka, Zambia. *World Journal of Advanced Research and Reviews (WJARR)*, *14*(3), pp.159-169.

Simuyaba, M., 2019. *Sickle cell disease associated co-morbidity with pneumonia outcomes among under-five children referred to university teaching hospital between 2011-2014 in Lusaka, Zambia* (Doctoral dissertation, The University of Zambia).

Sinkala, E., 2017. *Bacterial Translocation in Hepatosplenic Schistosomiasis Patients Seen at the University Teaching Hospital, Lusaka, Zambia* (Doctoral dissertation, University of Zambia).

Suali, L., Mohammad Salih, F.A., Ibrahim, M.Y., Jeffree, M.S.B., Thomas, F.M., Siew Moy, F., Shook Fe, Y., Suali, E., Sudi, S. and Sunggip, C., 2023. Genotype-Phenotype Study of β-Thalassemia Patients in Sabah. *Hemoglobin*, pp.1-8.

Telen, M.J., Malik, P. and Vercellotti, G.M., 2019. Therapeutic strategies for sickle cell disease: towards a multi-agent approach. *Nature reviews Drug discovery*, *18*(2), pp.139-158.

White, S., Foster, R., Marks, J., Morshead, R., Goldsmith, L., Barlow, S., Sin, J. and Gillard, S., 2020. The effectiveness of one-to-one peer support in mental health services: a systematic review and meta-analysis. *BMC psychiatry*, *20*(1), pp.1-20.

www.ingramcontent.com/pod-product-compliance
Lightning Source LLC
Chambersburg PA
CBHW051422290426
44109CB00016B/1392